MODERN MEDICINE
FOR THE MRCP

MODERN MEDICINE
FOR THE MRCP

KEVIN A. DAVIES
MA MD MRCP,
Senior Lecturer in Rheumatology and Medicine,
Royal Postgraduate Medical School,
Honorary Consultant Physician, Hammersmith Hospital

JUSTIN C. MASON
BSc MRCP,
Senior Registrar, Department of Medicine,
Hammersmith Hospital

WILLIAM A. LYNN
MD MRCP,
Consultant in Infectious Diseases and General Medicine,
Ealing Hospital,
Honorary Senior Lecturer, Hammersmith Hospital

TIMOTHY J. AITMAN
MRCP D.Phil,
Clinician Scientist, Molecular Medicine Group,
MRC Clinical Sciences Centre,
Honorary Senior Lecturer, RPMS,
Honorary Consultant Physician, Hammersmith Hospital

WB SAUNDERS COMPANY LTD
LONDON   PHILADELPHIA   TORONTO
SYDNEY   TOKYO

W.B. Saunders Company Ltd   24–28 Oval Road
London NW1 7DX

The Curtis Center
Independence Square West
Philadelphia, PA 19106-3399, USA

Harcourt Brace & Company
55 Horner Avenue
Toronto, Ontario M8Z 4X6, Canada

Harcourt Brace & Company, Australia
30–52 Smidmore Street
Marrickville, NSW 2204, Australia

Harcourt Brace & Company, Japan
Ichibancho Central Building,
22–1 Ichibancho
Chiyoda-ku, Tokyo 102, Japan

A catalogue record for this book is available from the British Library

ISBN 0–7020–2112–1

Typeset by LaserScript, Mitcham, Surrey
Printed and bound in Great Britain by
WBC Book Manufacturers, Bridgend, Mid Glamorgan

PREFACE

Medicine is a constantly developing speciality, and advances in basic scientific research are impinging more and more on our everyday clinical practice. For this reason, questions relating both to basic science as applied to clinical medicine, and to modern therapeutic and diagnostic methods are forming an increasingly important part of the MRCP examination, both in Part 1 and Part 2. Candidates are expected to be aware of recent developments in medicine published in journals such as the *Lancet, New England Journal of Medicine, BMJ* or *Quarterly Journal of Medicine.*

In this book we have provided 155 multiple choice questions; each consists of a stem with five possible responses that must be designated true or false by the student. These questions emphasise particular areas of contemporary medical and scientific interest such as genetics, molecular biology, therapeutics, infectious diseases (particularly HIV and AIDS) and immunology. Few of the topics addressed are adequately covered in standard textbooks.

The questions are not designed to be easy, and our recommendation is that readers tackle a maximum of ten questions at a time, attempt to answer them 'blind' – and then refer to the answers in the second part of the book. The answers and explanations are generally of MRCP standard or above, and as well as providing core knowledge which will be of use in an examination context, we hope that working through the book will stimulate readers to read more widely in areas which interest them, and in many instances provide practical information which will be of use in their day to day clinical practice. Certain topics (e.g. the biology of nitric oxide) are covered in more than one question, emphasising slightly different aspects of the subject. Do not be discouraged if you seem to score poorly at first! This book is designed both for self-assessment, and as a learning tool.

Kevin Davies

ACKNOWLEDGEMENTS

The authors thank Dr Simon Pearce (Molecular Endocrinology, MRC Clinical Sciences Centre) and Dr Kevin Talbot (Genetics Laboratory, Department of Biochemistry, University of Oxford) for assistance with the questions on molecular biology and genetics.

QUESTIONS

1. *Structure of HIV:*
   (a) p24 is a viral envelope protein.
   (b) The core contains two copies of the HIV RNA genome.
   (c) HIV may express host proteins on its surface.
   (d) Zidovudine inhibits reverse transcriptase encoded by the HIV *Rev* gene.
   (e) gp120 is encoded by the *Env* gene.

2. *Identification of disease genes by positional cloning:*
   (a) Requires some prior knowledge of the structure or function of the gene product.
   (b) Is not possible for polygenic disorders.
   (c) Is also known as 'reverse genetics'.
   (d) Initially requires linkage of an affected pedigree to a polymorphic genetic marker.
   (e) Was successful in the cloning of the cystic fibrosis gene.

3. *Complement and complement receptors:*
   (a) Genetic deficiency of classical pathway complement components is associated with the development of SLE.
   (b) An acquired reduction of erythrocyte complement receptor type 1 (CR1) is found in patients with lupus.
   (c) Deficiency of terminal pathway complement components results in increased frequency and severity of meningococcal meningitis.
   (d) Homozygous C1 inhibitor deficiency causes hereditary angio-oedema.
   (e) Regular monitoring of C3, C4 and haemolytic complement activity is useful in the management of SLE, microscopic polyarteritis and Wegener's granulomatosis.

4. *Viral hepatitis:*
   (a) Hepatitis A is an RNA virus.
   (b) Less than 10% of patients infected with hepatitis C develop chronic infection.
   (c) The delta virus requires co-infection with hepatitis B to produce disease.
   (d) Hepatitis E is transmitted by sexual contact or blood transfusion.
   (e) Hepatitis C infection is a cause of cryoglobulinaemia.

5. *Herpes virus infections:*
   (a) Human herpes virus type 6 (HHV6) is the causative agent of roseola infantum.
   (b) A herpes virus, HHV8, has been detected in HIV-associated Kaposi sarcoma lesions but not sporadic KS.
   (c) Herpes B virus is transmitted by monkeys.
   (d) Acyclovir is phosphorylated by a herpes virus thymidine kinase.
   (e) The anti-herpes drug foscarnet is a nucleoside analogue and acts by chain termination when incorporated into DNA.

6. *Cancer genetics:*
   (a) Loss of heterozygosity of a genetic marker in a tumour suggests that it may be close to a tumour suppressor gene.
   (b) Monoclonality of a tumour can be established using analysis of lyonisation (random X-chromosome inactivation) in a male.
   (c) Dominant cancer traits (such as retinoblastoma) require there to have been two somatic mutations to cause a tumour.
   (d) An individual tumour cannot be caused by both activation of an oncogene and inactivation of a tumour suppressor gene.
   (e) The function of most tumour suppressor genes is to regulate the cell cycle and cell division.

7. *Fas, apoptosis and the pathogenesis of SLE:*
   (a) Fas is a 43 kDa glycoprotein which is involved in inducing apoptosis only in B lymphocytes.
   (b) Up to 60% human subjects with lupus have elevated levels of soluble Fas protein in their serum.
   (c) Transcription of the *Fas* gene is defective in MRL/lpr lupus-prone mice, resulting in accelerated apoptosis of cells.
   (d) B-cell hyperactivity is a common feature of human SLE and the MRL/lpr murine lupus model.
   (e) Levels of Fas protein on the surface of B cells from peripheral blood in patients with SLE are reduced compared with those in normal subjects.

8. *Falciparum malaria:*
   (a) Intraerythrocytic schizonts are common.
   (b) Haemoglobin S heterozygotes (AS) are relatively protected.
   (c) The incubation period is 7–10 days.
   (d) Nephrotic syndrome is a complication.
   (e) CD31 is an endothelial cell receptor for *Plasmodium falciparum.*

9. *The following are true regarding opportunistic infections in patients with AIDS:*
   (a) *Bartonella (Rochalimea hensulae)* infection may present with skin lesions.
   (b) Fluconazole is suitable maintenance therapy for invasive aspergillosis.
   (c) Progressive multi-focal leucoencephalopathy is due to infection with a DNA polyoma virus.
   (d) *Cryptosporidium parvae* is a frequent cause of chronic diarrhoea.
   (e) Cytomegalovirus is a common cause of pneumonitis.

10. *Trinucleotide repeat elements in DNA:*
    (a) Are useful polymorphisms for disease linkage studies.
    (b) May cause Huntington's chorea if pathologically contracted.
    (c) Explain the phenomenon of anticipation seen in successive generations with myotonic dystrophy.
    (d) Have no known biological function.
    (e) Expansion may be associated with some cases of X-linked mental retardation.

11. *In Crohn's disease:*
    (a) pANCA are found in a distinct sub-group of patients.
    (b) There is an association with a rare allele of the intracellular adhesion molecule-1 (ICAM-1) gene.
    (c) An anti-erythrocyte antibody has also been described.
    (d) There is an association with the HLA class III genes and the TNF gene locus.
    (e) Anti-TNF monoclonal antibody therapy has been shown to be highly effective in some patients.

12. *Antiprotozoal drugs:*
    (a) Metronidazole is the drug of choice for acute amoebic dysentery.
    (b) Sodium stibogluconate is effective treatment for visceral leishmaniasis.
    (c) Tetracycline is the treatment of choice for trichomonas vaginalis.
    (d) *Toxoplasma gondii* infections are usually self-limiting.
    (e) Nebulised pentamidine is effective against *Pneumocystis carinii*.

13. *Gastrointestinal infections:*
    (a) *Cyclospora* spp. have recently been described as a cause of human diarrhoea.
    (b) *Clostridium difficile* only causes diarrhoea after antibiotic use.
    (c) Giardiasis has an associated eosinophilia in 30% of cases.
    (d) Enterohaemorrhagic *E. coli* may cause thrombocytopaenia.
    (e) *Bacillus cereus* causes diarrhoea 18–36 hours after ingestion.

14. *Mendelian inheritance:*
    (a) Implies that women cannot be affected by disease traits carried on the X-chromosome.
    (b) May be difficult to distinguish from a vertically transmitted infection.
    (c) Does not apply for mitochondrial genes.
    (d) Is usually assumed in a disease linkage study.
    (e) Has not occurred if a child has uniparental isodisomy.

15. *Nitric oxide:*
    (a) Is synonymous with endothelium-derived growth factor (EDGF).
    (b) Can be stimulated by longitudinal shear stress generated by blood flow within vessels.
    (c) May be produced by the endothelium as a consequence of NO synthase activity in response to bradykinin, acetylcholine, and 5-hydroxytryptamine.
    (d) Stimulates platelet adhesion and aggregation within the vessel.
    (e) In the heart, NO reduces ventricular compliance in diastole and increases the duration of contraction, in addition to markedly depressing systolic contraction.

16. *Antihelminthic drugs; the following are correctly paired:*
    (a) Threadworms : mebendazole.
    (b) *Taenia solium* : thiabendazole.
    (c) *Ascaris lumbricoides* : levamisole.
    (d) Filiariasis : diethylcarbamazine.
    (e) *Strongyloides stercoralis* : niclosamide.

17. *Bacteria:*
    (a) Lipopolysaccharide is found in the inner membrane of Gram-negative bacilli.
    (b) Fluorescent staining with auramine can be used to detect pneumocystis in bronchial lavage specimens.
    (c) *Listeria monocytogenes* is a Gram-negative rod.
    (d) *Staphylococcus aureus* is coagulase positive.
    (e) Cryptosporidiosis can be diagnosed by unstained stool microscopy.

18. *Alzheimer's disease:*
    (a) Accumulation of magnesium may contribute to disease pathogenesis.
    (b) Alleles of the gene for apolipoprotein E are associated with up to a 15-fold increased risk of late onset disease.
    (c) Early onset disease frequently shows recessive inheritance.
    (d) Early onset Alzheimer's disease may be predicted by DNA sequence analysis in affected pedigrees.
    (e) Patients with Down's syndrome characteristically develop Alzheimer's disease in their early 40s.

19. *Anti-neutrophil cytoplasmic antibodies:*
    (a) May be detectable by indirect immunofluorescence in patients with SLE.
    (b) Anti-proteinase 3 antibodies are strongly associated with Wegener's granulomatosis.
    (c) Anti-myeloperoxidase antibodies occur in microscopic polyangiitis.
    (d) Usually fall with therapy.
    (e) Have little value in predicting relapse in systemic vasculitis.

20. *Lyme disease:*
    (a) Is a flea-borne disease.
    (b) Cranial nerve palsy is a complication.
    (c) Joints are involved in up to 80% of patients.
    (d) Cardiac involvement is seen in 40% of patients.
    (e) Metronidazole is the treatment of choice.

21. *Communicable diseases:*
    (a) Notification is the responsibility of the microbiology laboratory.
    (b) HIV is a notifiable disease.
    (c) Failure to report a notifiable disease is an offence.
    (d) Syphilis is a notifiable disease.
    (e) Patients with tuberculosis can be detained and treated against their will.

22. *The polymerase chain reaction:*
    (a) Requires the presence of multiple copies of the DNA template.
    (b) Under standard conditions results in the production of a single-stranded product.
    (c) Can be used to diagnose herpes simplex encephalitis from CSF.
    (d) Can be used to perform prenatal diagnosis on a single embryo cell.
    (e) Requires no knowledge of the DNA sequence of the template to be amplified.

23. *Xenotransplantation:*
    (a) The major target antigen is a disaccharide expressed in some monkeys, pigs and lower mammals, but not in humans.
    (b) T cell-mediated immediate rejection is a major problem.
    (c) Genetic modification of complement control proteins in the donor tissue can modify the hyperacute rejection process.
    (d) Is hindered by the presence of naturally-occurring xenoreactive antibodies in the donor.
    (e) Rejection may potentially be reduced by enzymatic remodelling of donor carbohydrate antigens to resemble human blood group molecules.

24. *Plasma exchange:*
    (a) Requires anti-coagulation during the procedure.
    (b) Is used in the treatment of anti-GBM disease.
    (c) Is of proven value in the long-term management of lupus nephritis.
    (d) Is contraindicated in patients with cryoglobulinaemia.
    (e) May cause a fall in platelet count.

25. *The kidney:*
    (a) Renal blood flow is mainly distributed to the medulla.
    (b) Non-steroidal anti-inflammatory drugs increase renal blood flow.
    (c) Renal plasma flow varies significantly with systemic arterial blood pressure.
    (d) Angiotensin II dilates the efferent arteriole.
    (e) Measurement of urea clearance may over-estimate the true GFR.

26. *Rheumatic syndromes associated with HIV infection:*
    (a) Reiter's syndrome.
    (b) Crystal arthropathy.
    (c) Sjögren's syndrome.
    (d) Still's disease.
    (e) Seronegative polyarthritis.

27. *Corticosteroids are beneficial in:*
    (a) Childhood meningitis.
    (b) Tuberculous meningitis.
    (c) Cerebral malaria.
    (d) Typhoid fever.
    (e) Septic shock.

28. *The use of thrombolytic therapy following myocardial infarction is absolutely contraindicated:*
    (a) After a liver biopsy 2 weeks previously.
    (b) In patients with a previous history of streptococcal infection.
    (c) After a cerebrovascular accident in the previous 6 months.
    (d) In early pregnancy.
    (e) In a diabetic patient with proliferative retinopathy.

29. *Gilbert's syndrome:*
    (a) Usually carries the risk of severe liver disease in later life.
    (b) Is characteristically due to reduced hepatic bilirubin UDP-glucuronyl transferase (UDPGT) activity.
    (c) May be due to defect(s) in the promoter region of the disease gene.
    (d) Is characterised by conjugated hyperbilirubinaemia.
    (e) Results in decreases in serum bilirubin levels after food.

30. *Killed vaccines are:*
    (a) Pertussis.
    (b) Yellow fever.
    (c) Rubella.
    (d) Polio.
    (e) Chicken pox.

31. *Cyclooxygenase (COX):*
    (a) COX-1 is the predominant isoform involved in the inflammatory response.
    (b) COX-2 is an inducible isoform.
    (c) COX-2 is the predominant isoform involved in synthesis of prostaglandins.
    (d) Nabumetone is predominantly a COX-1 synthesis inhibitor.
    (e) COX-1 is the predominant isoform involved in the anti-thrombotic effect of aspirin.

32. *Patients with AIDS:*
   (a) Following infection with HIV, AIDS develops at a median of 3–5 years.
   (b) Candidaemia is a frequent complication.
   (c) Reactivation of toxoplasmosis often presents with choroidoretinitis.
   (d) Cryptococcosis is commoner in African patients.
   (e) Thrombocytopaenia is the result of bone marrow suppression.

33. *Anti-retroviral drugs:*
   (a) Combining zidovudine (AZT) with didanosine (DDI) results in significantly enhanced patient survival.
   (b) Zidovudine inhibits the replication of HIV and HTLV-1.
   (c) Pancreatitis is the major side-effect of zalcitadine (DDC).
   (d) Treatment with zidovudine during pregnancy reduces mother–child transmission of HIV.
   (e) Resistance of HIV to zidovudine is due to the failure of zidovudine to penetrate infected cells.

34. *Mitochondrial DNA:*
   (a) Mutations have been implicated in diabetes mellitus.
   (b) In humans 70% is inherited from the mother.
   (c) Shows heteroplasmy.
   (d) Is circular.
   (e) Mutations show a poor correlation with disease severity.

35. *Gene therapy for human disease:*
   (a) Has to date mainly been aimed at the correction of monogenic defects in germ cells prior to fertilisation.
   (b) Has been successfully used to improve immune function in adenosine deaminase deficiency in affected children.
   (c) Retroviral vectors for gene therapy of human disease are not used because these vectors encode the gene for reverse transcriptase.
   (d) Mounting an immune response against replaced proteins is unlikely to happen in gene therapy because recipients will always have had some level of expression of the deficient protein in early infancy.
   (e) Gene therapy for cystic fibrosis or sickle cell disease cannot succeed because most affected patients have identical mutations in both copies of their disease genes.

36. *Complement receptor type 1 (CR1):*
    (a) Is found only on red blood cells in primates.
    (b) Receptor numbers on erythrocytes vary in the normal population.
    (c) Is involved in the processing of immune complexes.
    (d) Is a co-factor for the inactivation of C3.
    (e) In soluble form has been shown experimentally to reduce the severity of reperfusion-induced myocardial injury.

37. *Acute intermittent porphyria:*
    (a) Is commoner in females.
    (b) Causes a motor neuropathy.
    (c) Causes elevation of porphobilinogen and δ-aminolaevulinic acid in urine.
    (d) May be precipitated by alcohol.
    (e) Commonly presents in childhood.

38. *Amyloidosis:*
    (a) Is characterised by the intracellular deposition of autologous protein in the form of amyloid fibrils.
    (b) Familial amyloid polyneuropathy is generally associated with single amino acid variants of plasma transthyretin.
    (c) Structural abnormalities of apolipoprotein A1 (apoA1), the major apolipoprotein of LDL, are also associated with amyloid.
    (d) Amyloid occurring secondary to a persistent acute phase response may regress with anti-inflammatory and immunosuppressive therapy.
    (e) May be diagnosed by the injection of radiolabelled serum amyloid P component, and gamma-scintigraphy.

39. *Prion diseases:*
    (a) Are caused by a transmissible agent.
    (b) Have a short incubation period.
    (c) Produce a slowly progressive dementia.
    (d) Are a recognised cause of a familial form of ataxia.
    (e) May be transmitted as a complication of organ transplantation.

40. *Systemic sclerosis:*
    (a) Hypertension is rarely seen.
    (b) Antibodies to Scl 70 are a feature.
    (c) Methotrexate retards disease expression.
    (d) Raised titres of anti-endothelial cell antibodies are found.
    (e) Raynaud's phenomenon may precede skin involvement by some years.

41. *Schistosomiasis:*
    (a) *S. haematobium* eggs may be found in rectal biopsies.
    (b) Is the cause of Katayama fever.
    (c) Is a cause of granulomatous hepatitis.
    (d) May present with paraplegia.
    (e) Albendazole is the treatment of choice.

42. *Genomic imprinting:*
    (a) May be caused by DNA methylation.
    (b) Occurs only in primates.
    (c) May explain the mode of inheritance in Prader–Willi syndrome.
    (d) May explain random inactivation of paternal or maternal genes.
    (e) Can explain sex-linked inheritance in muscular dystrophy.

43. *Drugs causing cholestatic jaundice:*
    (a) Methotrexate.
    (b) Tetracycline.
    (c) Chlopromazine.
    (d) Isoniazid.
    (e) Nitrofurantoin.

44. *The ratio between CD4 and CD8 T cells:*
    (a) Varies little between normal subjects.
    (b) Is high in patients with acute viral diseases, allograft rejection and haemophilia.
    (c) Is useful in monitoring patients infected with HIV who develop AIDS.
    (d) Is generally lower in normal males than in females.
    (e) Increases with age.

45. *Vasculitis:*
    (a) Is associated with parvovirus B19 infection.
    (b) A positive anti-neutrophil cytoplasmic test is invariably seen.
    (c) C-reactive protein levels may reflect disease activity.
    (d) Is associated with HIV infection.
    (e) Is confined to medium-sized and small arteries.

46. *Viral hepatitis:*
    (a) Hepatitis E is transmitted by the parenteral route.
    (b) 10–20% of patients with hepatitis C will progress to chronic liver disease.
    (c) Hepatitis D has an RNA core with an outer envelope composed of hepatitis B surface antigen.
    (d) Interferon-γ is indicated in chronic hepatitis B infection.
    (e) Hepatitis C has a circular RNA genome.

47. *Infections due to mycobacteria:*
    (a) Lepromatous leprosy is associated with impaired cell-mediated immunity.
    (b) Interferon-γ enhances intracellular killing of mycobacteria.
    (c) BCG vaccination affords protection against leprosy.
    (d) Tuberculous meningitis is more frequent and often resistant to therapy in patients co-infected with HIV.
    (e) Corticosteroids should be avoided in patients with active tuberculosis.

48. *Hypertrophic cardiomyopathy:*
    (a) Causes progressive myocardial hypertrophy during the first two decades of life.
    (b) When familial, is inherited as an autosomal recessive disease.
    (c) May be caused by mutations in the myocardial sarcomere proteins myosin, tropomyosin and troponin.
    (d) May cause syncopal attacks and sudden death in early adult life.
    (e) A jerky radial pulse may distinguish this condition from valvular aortic stenosis.

49. *Cystic fibrosis:*
    (a) Is an autosomal recessive disorder.
    (b) Is due to a mutation of the cystic fibrosis transmembrane conductance regulator (CFTR) gene.
    (c) In mild form, may result in the congenital absence of the vas deferens.
    (d) Is associated with reduced sweat chloride concentrations, due to a defect in the cAMP-regulated chloride channel on the apical surface of epithelial cells.
    (e) May be amenable to gene therapy using liposome vectors.

50. *HIV-1-associated neurological disease:*
    (a) Affects 40–60% patients with AIDS.
    (b) Is the commonest cause of dementia in young American males.
    (c) Typically results in an encephalopathic illness in affected children.
    (d) May result from direct infection of microglial cells, brain macrophages, oligodendrocytes and neurones by HIV-1, and the production of toxic viral structural proteins within these cells.
    (e) May be associated with high levels of TNF-α expression within the CNS.

51. *Mannose binding protein:*
    (a) Is structurally similar to complement components C1q and C3.
    (b) Is synthesised by hepatocytes.
    (c) Activates complement by both the classical and alternative pathways.
    (d) Is found at low levels in some individuals, which results in an immunodeficiency syndrome.
    (e) Is an acute phase protein.

52. *Hepatitis C:*
    (a) Is a DNA virus.
    (b) Diagnosis is based on immunoblotting hepatitis C antigens present in infected serum.
    (c) The route of infection is unclear in 30% of patients.
    (d) Can be transmitted by saliva and sexual intercourse.
    (e) Mother to infant transmission does not occur.

53. *Polycythaemia:*
   (a) Haemoglobin concentration is the best measure of reponse to treatment.
   (b) A red cell mass greater than 100% is diagnostic.
   (c) Thrombosis is a side-effect associated with regular venesection.
   (d) Hydroxyurea is the most commonly used cytotoxic agent used in the treatment of primary proliferative polycythaemia.
   (e) Uterine leiomyomata are a recognised cause.

54. *Progression of HIV infection:*
   (a) With disease progression HIV-associated lymphadenopathy becomes more prominent.
   (b) Serum neopterin is a marker of macrophage activation and is predictive of progression to AIDS.
   (c) Syncytia-inducing strains of HIV are associated with rapid disease progression.
   (d) Active infection with hepatitis B leads to increased HIV replication.
   (e) Smoking is associated with a worse prognosis.

55. *HLA-B27:*
   (a) Is associated with ankylosing spondylitis, acute anterior uveitis, and infective arthritis caused by *Chlamydia* and certain Gram-negative organisms.
   (b) Occurs more frequently in males with seronegative arthritides.
   (c) Is associated with more severe disease when it occurs as part of an extended haplotype incorporating certain TNF alleles.
   (d) Is involved in the presentation of peptides of 30–40 amino acids to CD8 positive cytotoxic T lymphocytes.
   (e) Causes a multi-system inflammatory disease when introduced transgenically into rats in association with β_2-microglobulin.

56. *The following typically occur in homocystinuria:*
   (a) Upward lens dislocation.
   (b) Thromboses.
   (c) Seizures.
   (d) Aortic incompetence.
   (e) Learning difficulties.

57. *Atherogenesis:*
    (a) The tunica media is the site of plaque formation.
    (b) Smooth muscle proliferation is a central feature.
    (c) NK cells migrating into the intima are involved in plaque formation.
    (d) Low-density lipoproteins induce endothelial cell activation.
    (e) Plaque formation is induced by laminar flow close to arterial branches.

58. *The rheumatoid joint:*
    (a) IL-1 and TNF stimulate synthesis of metalloproteinases by chondrocytes and macrophages.
    (b) Interferon-γ is found in high concentration in synovial fluid.
    (c) Transforming growth factor-β has a regulatory role.
    (d) In chronic rheumatoid arthritis synovial fluid T cells are predominantly of the memory subtype.
    (e) The IL-1 receptor antagonist is not found.

59. *Syphilis:*
    (a) Lymphadenopathy is seen in secondary rather than primary disease.
    (b) Central nervous system invasion commonly occurs in secondary syphilis.
    (c) Erythromycin is suitable therapy for secondary syphilis in pregnancy.
    (d) False-positive TPHA may occur in pregnancy.
    (e) Obliterative endarteritis is a characteristic pathological finding.

60. *Genetics of diabetes mellitus:*
    (a) HLA is the major genetic influence on development of type 1 (insulin-dependent) diabetes.
    (b) Insulin receptor defects may cause extreme insulin resistance and congenital cranial dysmorphism.
    (c) Insulin receptor defects are a common cause of non-insulin dependent diabetes.
    (d) Defects in the glucokinase gene cause 50–60% of cases of maturity onset diabetes of the young (MODY).
    (e) Mutations in mitochondrial DNA account for up to 5% of cases of maternally inherited diabetes.

61. *Anti-nuclear antibodies:*
    (a) Anti–Sm antibodies are present in 80% of patients with systemic lupus erythematosus.
    (b) The Jo-1 antigen is a tRNA histidyl synthetase.
    (c) Anti-centromere antibodies are typically found in mixed connective tissue disease.
    (d) Anti-RNP antibodies are found in 40% of patients with systemic sclerosis.
    (e) Anti–La antibodies are strongly associated with fetal congenital heart block.

62. *During seroconversion to HIV-1:*
    (a) There is an acute fall of both CD4 and CD8 lymphocytes.
    (b) Patients are more infectious.
    (c) Anti-HIV antibodies are not detectable until 6–12 weeks after the onset of symptoms.
    (d) A cytotoxic lymphocyte response against HIV infected cells appears before detectable HIV-specific antibodies.
    (e) Patients with asymptomatic primary infection are more likely to develop AIDS within 3 years than patients with symptomatic illness.

63. *Nitric oxide:*
    (a) Is a neurotransmitter.
    (b) Can be induced by cytokines.
    (c) Facilitates platelet aggregation.
    (d) Can be infused intravenously in the treatment of unstable angina.
    (e) Acts by causing a rise in cyclic GMP (guanosine monophosphate).

64. *Familial mediterranean fever:*
    (a) Usually presents in childhood.
    (b) Is common in Jews and Armenians.
    (c) Most commonly presents with abdominal pain.
    (d) Attacks usually last for 1–2 days only.
    (e) Is associated with elevated IL-6 levels, an elevation in CRP, and a pre-disposition to amyloid.

65. *Sulphasalazine:*
    (a) Is useful in the management of rheumatoid arthritis.
    (b) Is contraindicated in elderly patients.
    (c) May cause thrombocytopenia.
    (d) Can cause a lupus-like syndrome.
    (e) May result in the staining of soft contact lenses.

66. *HLA and disease:*
    (a) Primary Sjögrens syndrome is associated with HLA DR3, B8, DQ2 and the C4A null gene.
    (b) Rheumatoid arthritis is associated with HLA DR2.
    (c) Behçets syndrome is associated with HLA DRw52.
    (d) Goodpasture's syndrome is associated with HLA DR4.
    (e) Pemphigus vulgaris is associated with HLA DR4.

67. *Whipple's disease:*
    (a) Is the result of infection with *Tropheryma whippelii.*
    (b) The polymerase chain reaction has formed the basis of a diagnostic test for Whipple's disease.
    (c) Is a cause of ophthalmoplegia and dementia.
    (d) Treatment for up to a year with co-trimoxazole is recommended to prevent relapse.
    (e) Is classically associated with a positive periodic acid Schiff test.

68. *Varicella-zoster infections:*
    (a) Trigeminal shingles may be complicated by contralateral hemiplegia.
    (b) Topical corticosteroids are used in cases with corneal involvement.
    (c) Following primary infection the virus enters a latent state in the motor nerve roots.
    (d) Chickenpox pneumonia is commoner in childhood.
    (e) Primary infection can be prevented with hyperimmune globulin up to 6 days following exposure.

69. *Cystic fibrosis genetics:*
    (a) Approximately 70% of mutant alleles are accounted for by the same 3 base pair deletion.
    (b) The cystic fibrosis gene encodes a transmembrane protein regulating chloride transport.
    (c) Antenatal screening for the disorder is not possible because the disease gene is not expressed in fetal tissue.
    (d) One in 25 of the population are heterozygotes for the cystic fibrosis mutation.
    (e) Successive generations are not generally affected because inheritance is autosomal recessive.

70. *Immunophilins:*
    (a) Are proteins which serve as receptors for certain immunosuppressive drugs.
    (b) Levels are very low in the nervous system.
    (c) Are mainly of high molecular weight.
    (d) Are linked to a number of different intracellular transduction systems, many of which are calcium-dependent.
    (e) May affect IL-2 gene expression.

71. *Low molecular weight heparins:*
    (a) May be taken by mouth.
    (b) May be given once daily.
    (c) Are best monitored by the APTT.
    (d) Are best monitored by the PT.
    (e) Have a more predictable dose–response relationship than conventional non-fractionated heparins.

72. *Sjögrens syndrome:*
    (a) Commonly complicates graft versus host disease.
    (b) Is associated with antibodies against the Ro but not the La antigen.
    (c) May be complicated by renal tubular acidosis type 1.
    (d) Glandular destruction is mediated by CD8 positive T lymphocytes.
    (e) Is associated with a hypogammaglobulinaemia.

73. *Immunodeficiency syndromes:*
    (a) Bruton's agammaglobulinaemia is the result of an autosomal recessive defect.
    (b) DiGeorge syndrome results in an absence of T cells due to thymic aplasia.
    (c) Wiskott–Aldrich syndrome results in susceptibility to encapsulated extracellular bacteria.
    (d) Bare lymphocyte syndrome is a lack of MHC class I expression.
    (e) Adenosine deaminase deficiency results in a severe combined immunodeficiency phenotype.

74. *HIV:*
    (a) HIV-1 is a retrovirus infection from the Flaviviridae family of RNA viruses.
    (b) Most cases of HIV-2 are associated with West Africa.
    (c) HIV RNA is incorporated into the human genome to cause persistent infection.
    (d) Changes in the V3 subregion of the HIV envelope alters the cellular tropism of the virus.
    (e) HIV protease inhibitors prevent viral replication by blocking integration of HIV into host DNA.

75. *Antenatal diagnosis of genetic disease:*
    (a) RFLP analysis can be used to detect disorders where the genetic defect has been characterised.
    (b) Requires previous DNA analysis of affected family members if gene sequence analysis is to be employed.
    (c) Genetic recombination can cause false-positive results.
    (d) Chorionic villus sampling can be carried out at 12 weeks of gestation.
    (e) Can be used to detect cases of Huntington's chorea.

76. *Sub-acute sclerosing panencephalitis (SSPE):*
    (a) May be associated with early and often extensive involvement of the visual system, including chorioretinitis, optic atrophy, cortical blindness and papilloedema.
    (b) Occurs three to four times more commonly in girls.
    (c) Is thought to be due to a latent CNS infection with measles virus, and is associated with measles antibody in the CSF, but rarely in the serum.
    (d) Is more likely to develop in children who contract measles in late childhood.
    (e) Has fallen in frequency with the widespread use of measles vaccination.

77. *The following auto-antibodies are correctly paired with their disease:*
    (a) Anti-smooth muscle and primary biliary cirrhosis.
    (b) Anti-Sm and polymyositis.
    (c) Anti-RNP and primary Sjögren's syndrome.
    (d) Anti-centromere and CREST syndrome.
    (e) Anti-I and cold agglutinin disease.

78. *A 30-year-old man returning from the tropics presents with explosive diarrhoea, weight loss and glossitis:*
    (a) Giardiasis is a likely diagnosis.
    (b) Intestinal biopsy and sampling would be helpful.
    (c) Barium enema is a useful investigation.
    (d) Folate deficiency may be an associate.
    (e) Typhoid is a likely diagnosis.

79. *Antibiotics that inhibit protein synthesis by binding to ribosomes:*
    (a) Tetracycline.
    (b) Teicoplanin.
    (c) Ciprofloxacin.
    (d) Rifampicin.
    (e) Imipenem.

80. *Apoptosis:*
    (a) Is characterised by the release of free radicals.
    (b) The histopathological hallmark is cellular swelling.
    (c) Is responsible for the death of approximately 50% of all CNS neurones in embryogenesis.
    (d) Of tumour cells due to DNA damage is suppressed by mutation of the p53 gene product.
    (e) Requires the synthesis of new mRNA.

81. *Alzheimer's disease:*
    (a) There are around half a million diagnosed cases in the UK.
    (b) There is a strong association between the possession of the *APOE* gene ε4 and the development of the disease.
    (c) *APP* (amyloid precursor protein gene) on chromosome 21 codes for the β-amyloid-precursor protein, from which a peptide (β-amyloid peptide) is generated, which is deposited in the diseased brain.
    (d) Patients with Down's syndrome are at increased risk of developing the disease at a young age.
    (e) Tacrine may be of value in the disease by reducing the accumulation of precursor proteins in senile plaques.

82. *Inflammation:*
    (a) Acute inflammation is characterised by formation of an exudate.
    (b) Synovial infiltration with mononuclear cells is characteristically seen in gout.
    (c) Neutrophils predominate in chronic inflammatory lesions.
    (d) Granulomas are a feature of primary biliary cirrhosis.
    (e) Type IV hypersensitivity is an acute inflammatory reaction.

83. *T lymphocytes:*
    (a) Are all CD3 positive.
    (b) Are all CD4 positive.
    (c) Memory T cells are CD45Ro positive.
    (d) Produce interleukin-1 as their major lymphokine.
    (e) Are important in type 1 hypersensitivity reactions.

84. *Features of atypical pneumonia:*
    (a) *Legionella pneumophilia* typically induces a neutrophil leucocytosis.
    (b) Smokers are more likely to have experienced legionella infection.
    (c) *Mycoplasma pneumoniae* is an intracellular pathogen.
    (d) Mycoplasma infections are increased in the elderly.
    (e) *Coxiella burnetti* is the causative agent of Q fever.

85. *G-proteins:*
    (a) Are activated by the binding of an extracellular ligand to a membrane receptor.
    (b) Can be mutated in tumour cells.
    (c) Mediate the action of glucocorticoid hormones.
    (d) The $G_S\alpha$ subunit is inactivated by cholera toxin.
    (e) Bind to DNA to regulate gene transcription.

86. *Receptors:*
    (a) Particulate guanylate cyclase is a receptor for atrial naturetic peptide.
    (b) Drugs which open potassium channels cause vasoconstriction in man.
    (c) The main angiotensin II receptor in myocardial tissue is the AT_1 sub-type.
    (d) Antagonists of angiotensin II receptors (AT_1 sub-type) cause a rise in plasma angiotensin II levels.
    (e) Endothelin-1 is a potent vasodilator, and has mitogenic properties.

87. *Lymphocyte migration:*
    (a) Naive T cells localise in secondary lymphoid organs.
    (b) Memory T cells are larger than naive T cells.
    (c) Memory T cells preferentially migrate to non-lymphoid tissues.
    (d) T cells express surface L-selectin.
    (e) T cells migrate into lymph nodes across small arterioles.

88. *Mechanisms of action of bacterial toxins:*
    (a) The A subunit of cholera enterotoxin mediates entry of the toxin into the cell.
    (b) Diptheria toxin inhibits protein synthesis by blocking tRNA/mRNA interactions.
    (c) *Clostridium botulinum* neurotoxin antagonises the action of acetyl choline.
    (d) Pertussis toxin inhibits protein kinase C.
    (e) Toxic shock syndrome toxin 1 (TSST-1) is a super-antigen.

89. *Trinucleotide repeat expansions:*
    (a) Only cause neurodegenerative disease if they contain more than 200 repeat units.
    (b) Prevent expression of the Huntington disease gene.
    (c) Are stable in mitosis.
    (d) Provide an explanation for the phenomenon of genetic anticipation.
    (e) Is responsible for mental retardation due to the Fragile X syndrome.

90. *Hereditary haemorrhagic telangectasia:*
    (a) Displays great variability in severity between affected patients in the same family.
    (b) Is autosomally recessive.
    (c) Is associated with an increased risk of developing life-threatening pulmonary AVMs during pregnancy.
    (d) Is associated with mutations in the plasma protein endoglin.
    (e) Is associated with an increased risk of spontaneous abortion in affected pregnant women.

91. *Endothelial cells:*
    (a) Form a passive barrier between the circulation and the extracellular space.
    (b) May be activated by cytokines.
    (c) Can produce tumour necrosis factor (TNF).
    (d) Are functionally heterogeneous.
    (e) Play a central role in hyperacute graft rejection.

92. *Diseases and causative organisms:*
    (a) Erythema infectiosum (slapped cheek): Parvovirus B19.
    (b) Chagas' disease: *Leishmania brazilensis.*
    (c) Lyme disease: *Borrelia recurrentis.*
    (d) Lymphogranuloma venereum: *Haemophilus ducreyi.*
    (e) Rat bite fever *Streptobacillus moniliformis.*

93. *Genetic forms of dwarfism:*
    (a) Are most commonly caused by defects in the growth hormone and growth hormone receptor gene.
    (b) Due to growth hormone receptor mutations may be successfully treated with insulin-like growth factor-I.
    (c) If dominantly inherited may be due to achondroplasia.
    (d) Most cases of achondroplasia are caused by an identical mutation in the gene for a fibroblast growth factor receptor, FGFR3.
    (e) Cannot be due to achondroplasia if the patient is of normal intelligence.

94. *Neuropharmacology:*
    (a) The anti-emetic ondansetron is a serotonin uptake inhibitor.
    (b) Nomifensine inhibits dopamine uptake.
    (c) Monoamine oxidase inhibitors should not be co-administered with selective serotonin re-uptake inhibitors.
    (d) Tacrine does not cross the blood–brain barrier.
    (e) Sumatriptan is an agonist for 5-HT type 1 receptors, and is safe in patients with a history of ischaemic heart disease.

95. *Immune-mediated hypersensitivity:*
    (a) Type 1 reactions are IgE-mediated and are typically directed against antigens which enter through epithelial surfaces.
    (b) Type 2 reactions are mediated by immune complexes.
    (c) Type 2 reactions are generally mediated by complement-fixing antibodies.
    (d) Type 3 hypersensitivity is an aetiologic factor in the Dengue haemorrhagic shock syndrome which typically develops in pre-sensitised individuals.
    (e) Antibody and complement are necessary for the development of type 4 (delayed) hypersensitivity reactions.

96. *Twins:*
    (a) Comparison of concordance rates for a particular trait in dizygotic and monozygotic twins is commonly used in medical genetics to assess the relative effects of genetic and environmental factors.
    (b) Monozygotic twins result from a single zygote that divides into two separate embryos between 8 and 14 days after fertilization.
    (c) Monozygotic twins have a single chorion with a common circulation in over 90% cases.
    (d) Dizygotic twinning is familial.
    (e) The incidence of dizygotic and monozygotic twinning is much the same in all populations studied.

97. *Endothelial cell activation during inflammatory processes:*
    (a) Results in increased vascular permeability.
    (b) May result in the expression of class II MHC on endothelial cells.
    (c) Results in the production of nitric oxide.
    (d) Promotes the formation of an anticoagulant endothelial surface.
    (e) Induces endothelial cell shape change.

98. *Cytokines:*
    (a) Are low molecular weight glycoproteins.
    (b) IL-1, TNF and IL-6 are monocyte-derived cytokines.
    (c) Interferon-γ (IFN-γ) increases monocyte MHC class II expression.
    (d) IFN-γ is predominantly a fibroblast product.
    (e) A systemic vascular leak syndrome is a side-effect of treatment with IL-2.

99. *Malaria:*
    (a) *Plasmodium malariae* does not require primaquine to prevent relapse.
    (b) *P. vivax* enters erythrocytes after interaction with the Duffy antigen.
    (c) *P. falciparum* can only infect young erythrocytes.
    (d) Nephrotic syndrome is a complication of *P. malariae* but not other species of malaria.
    (e) If gametocytes are seen on blood films following therapy further treatment is not needed.

100. *Obesity in humans:*
    (a) Is commonly inherited as a Mendelian trait.
    (b) Is frequently caused by deficient leptin production.
    (c) Is associated with raised blood leptin concentration.
    (d) When associated with mental retardation may be due to Prader–Willi syndrome.
    (e) Is the predominant cause of hyperglycaemia in maturity-onset diabetes in the young (MODY).

101. *Non-steroidal anti-inflammatory drugs:*
    (a) Ibuprofen is generally associated with fewer gastrointestinal side-effects than other NSAIDs.
    (b) Azapropazone is one of the first drugs of choice in an elderly patient with acute gout.
    (c) Diclofenac may cause a biochemical hepatitis in patients with rheumatoid arthritis.
    (d) Tenoxicam is particularly useful for the therapy of acute gout, and is useful in the long-term management of patients with severe osteoarthritis of the hips.
    (e) Phenylbutazone is the drug of choice for the management of ankylosing spondylitis.

102. *Factor V_{Leiden}:*
    (a) Factor V_{Leiden} is an abnormal Factor V variant which causes resistance to the activity of protein C.
    (b) The mutation is due to the substitution of Arg by Gln at position 506.
    (c) The mutation occurs in 15% of normal subjects.
    (d) Factor V_{Leiden} is associated with an increased risk of thrombosis in patients taking the oral contraceptive pill.
    (e) The mutation cannot be detected by PCR-based methods when patients are taking oral anti-coagulants.

103. *Cytokines in disease:*
    (a) IL-1 is implicated in the induction of an acute phase response.
    (b) IL-6 is raised in giant cell arteritis.
    (c) Raised IL-6 results in a high CRP, anaemia and thrombocytopaenia.
    (d) Anti-TNF antibodies are effective in rheumatoid arthritis.
    (e) Treatment with soluble TNF-receptors may reduce morbidity and mortality in septic shock.

104. *Causes of erythema nodosum:*
    (a) Histoplasmosis.
    (b) Leprosy.
    (c) Pontiac fever.
    (d) Reactivation of tuberculosis.
    (e) Staphylococcal infections.

105. *Gaucher's disease:*
    (a) Shows dominant inheritance.
    (b) Is caused by an inherited defect in the lysosomal enzyme glucocerebrosidase.
    (c) Causes amyloid deposition in multiple organs.
    (d) The prevalence is increased among Ashkenazi Jews.
    (e) The carrier state may be diagnosed by molecular genetic analysis.

106. *Hepatitis B vaccination:*
    (a) Is indicated in health care workers who are likely to come into regular contact with patients or their body fluids.
    (b) Should be administered by sub-cutaneous injection.
    (c) Is indicated in i.v. drug abusers who are known to be hepatitis B surface antigen positive.
    (d) Confers adequate protection in 90% subjects within one month of administration.
    (e) Is less effective in elderly patients and renal patients receiving long-term haemodialysis.

107. *Cellular adhesion molecules:*
    (a) The integrins are single chain glycoproteins.
    (b) Intercellular adhesion molecule-1 (ICAM-1) is a receptor for both the rhinoviruses and the *Plasmodium falciparum* malarial parasite.
    (c) ICAM-1 is involved in the interaction between T cells and involved in the interaction between antigen presenting cells.
    (d) Raised plasma vascular cell adhesion molecule-1 and ICAM-1 are found in rheumatoid arthritis.
    (e) The selectins mediate leukocyte tethering and rolling on endothelium.

108. *Members of the immunoglobulin superfamily:*
    (a) ICAM-1.
    (b) E selectin.
    (c) MHC class II.
    (d) CD2.
    (e) Vascular cell adhesion molecule-1.

109. *ACE inhibitors:*
    (a) ACE-inhibitors and β-blockers reduce plasma renin activity.
    (b) ACE-inhibitors reduce mortality in congestive cardiac failure.
    (c) Assessment of renal vein renin activity is a good predictor of response to captopril.
    (d) Losartan is a specific angiotensin-II receptor antagonist, but its use is limited in many patients by the development of a chronic cough.
    (e) ACE-inhibitors may be associated with symptoms and serological abnormalities which resemble those seen in SLE.

110. *The human reproductive system and sex chromosomes:*
    (a) Up to 6 weeks of embryologic development, the developing gonad, whether chromosomally XX or XY, is bipotential.
    (b) The development of male gonads is dependent on the presence of a Y chromosome, and a phenotypic male cannot occur with a 46 XX karyotype.
    (c) X inactivation normally occurs randomly within female somatic cells.
    (d) The commonest sex chromosome defects in live-born infants and fetuses are trisomic.
    (e) Patients with Klinefelter syndrome are phenotypically male and appear physically normal until puberty.

111. *Leukocyte adhesion deficiency:*
    (a) Commonly results in life threatening bacterial infections.
    (b) Is the result of an integrin deficiency.
    (c) Is characterised by a marked neutropenia.
    (d) Two separate types have now been described.
    (e) There is a marked failure of lymphocyte migration at inflammatory sites.

112. *Monoclonal antibodies:*
   (a) Bind specifically to a single antigen.
   (b) Are produced by the fusion of T lymphoblasts and plasma cells.
   (c) Are of the IgM subclass.
   (d) Can only be produced in mice.
   (e) Are structurally monovalent.

113. *Associations of viral infections:*
   (a) Adult B-cell lymphoma: HTLV-1.
   (b) Post transplantation lymphoma: Epstein–Barr virus.
   (c) Renal failure: Hantaan virus.
   (d) Chronic fatigue syndrome: Epstein–Barr virus.
   (e) Anal carcinoma: Papilloma virus.

114. *Routes of acquiring infection:*
   (a) Brucellosis: Unpasteurised milk.
   (b) Bartonellosis: Sandfly bite.
   (c) Aspergillosis: Smoking marijuana.
   (d) Dengue fever: Tick bite.
   (e) Amoebic meningitis: Fresh water swimming.

115. *Osler–Weber–Rendu disease:*
   (a) May be genetically determined, or acquired.
   (b) May be complicated by stroke and brain abscess.
   (c) Recurrent haemorrhages from the gastrointestinal tract are uncommon.
   (d) Embolisation of brain and lung lesions may be successful.
   (e) Has very low penetrance in offspring of affected individuals.

116. *Monoclonal antibodies successful in treating rheumatoid arthritis:*
   (a) Anti-TNF.
   (b) Anti-E-selectin.
   (c) Anti-ICAM-1.
   (d) Anti-CD4.
   (e) Anti-IFN-γ.

117. *Parasitic infections:*
    (a) Ancylostoma infections often cause an iron-deficiency anaemia.
    (b) IL-6 is important in inducing eosinophilia in parasitic infections.
    (c) Oncocerciasis is diagnosed by identifying microfilaiae in thin blood films.
    (d) Cystercicosis results from infection with *Taenia sagginatum* (pork tapeworm).
    (e) *Trichinella spiralis* is a cause of myositis.

118. *Neurodegenerative disease:*
    (a) Creutzfeld–Jacob disease, scrapie, kuru and bovine spongiform encephalopathy may all be caused by prion particles.
    (b) Prion particles are composed of nucleic acids and protein.
    (c) Creutzfeld–Jacob disease occurs most commonly in the second and third decades of life.
    (d) The infectious prion protein is a modified host protein that can form into amyloid.
    (e) The frequency of kuru is increasing worldwide.

119. *Glucose-6-phosphate dehydrogenase deficiency:*
    (a) Is a highly heterogenous genetic disorder and occurs frequently in the Mediterranean and in American blacks.
    (b) Only occurs in males.
    (c) Results in increased susceptibility of erythrocytes to oxidative damage as consequence of greatly reduced stability of the variant proteins within the cell.
    (d) Causes favism.
    (e) May result in severe hamolytic anaemia following the administration of primaquine, dapsone or sulphonamide antibiotics.

120. *Acetylation polymorphism:*
   (a) Phenotypically slow acetylators are genotypically homozygous or heterozygous for the abnormal gene.
   (b) The polymorphism was first discovered when patients with tuberculosis were treated with isoniazid.
   (c) Slow and fast inactivation phenotypes are due to two alleles of the enzyme arylamine N-acetyltransferase.
   (d) The slow acetylation phenotype occurs most frequently in the Asian population.
   (e) Acetylator status can be rapidly determined by analysis of a patient's urine after drinking a cup of coffee.

121. *Succinylcholine sensitivity:*
   (a) Causes malignant hyperthermia.
   (b) Is due to a genetic defect in a serum cholinesterase enzyme, which occurs with a frequency of 1:20 000 in European populations.
   (c) Generally occurs only in homozygotes for the abnormal enzyme variant.
   (d) May result in the need to ventilate a patient artificially for several hours after the administration of a single dose of suxamethonium.
   (e) Can be readily diagnosed in relatives of affected patients by measurement of serum cholinesterase levels.

122. *Apoptosis:*
   (a) Apoptotic cell death results in a form of cellular necrosis.
   (b) Nuclear fragmentation is a characteristic feature of apoptosis.
   (c) SLE is associated with the inhibition of apoptosis.
   (d) Hodgkin's lymphoma is associated with increased apoptosis.
   (e) Many chemotherapeutic drugs induce apoptosis.

123. *Gram-negative septic shock:*
   (a) The cardiac index is characteristically reduced.
   (b) Tissue oxygen extraction is impaired.
   (c) Systemic vascular resistance is low.
   (d) Echthyma gangrenosum suggests infection with *Pseudomonas aeruginosa*.
   (e) Plasma lactate is increased.

124. *Venous thromboembolism:*
    (a) Is common in patients with the lupus anticoagulant or antiphospholipid antibodies.
    (b) Is associated with a point mutation in the gene for factor V in up to 50% of cases of familial venous thromboses.
    (c) May be caused by inherited defects in either the natural anticoagulant, protein C, or its co-factor, protein S.
    (d) A cause for familial thrombophilia should be sought in patients under 40 years with thromboembolism.
    (e) Is associated with homocystinuria and hyperhomocysteinaemia.

125. *HLA:*
    (a) Class I genes comprise HLA-A, HLA-B and HLA-D, all of which are located on the short arm of chromosome 6.
    (b) A Class I antigen consists of two chains: a heavy chain encoded within the major histocompatibility complex, and a highly polymorphic polypeptide called β_2-microglobulin.
    (c) HLA-alleles are co-dominant, and are transmitted as a haplotype.
    (d) HLA-DR2 occurs in 15–20% of normal controls, but in over 95% patients with narcolepsy.
    (e) Type 1 diabetes, myasthenia gravis, SLE and rheumatoid arthritis are all commonly associated with HLA-DR3.

126. *Mechanisms of drug actions:*
    (a) Nimodipine is a calcium slow channel antagonist which acts selectively on larger arterioles (diameter > 200 µm) in the visceral circulation.
    (b) Nizatidine is potent histamine H_2-receptor antagonist, with some H_1-receptor antagonist activity.
    (c) The effects of Omeprazole are mediated through binding to the parietal cell proton pump H^+, K^+–ATPase.
    (d) Pamidronate is an amino-substituted bisphosphonate that inhibits bone resorption by osteoclasts.
    (e) Acyclovir is preferentially phosphorylated in cells infected with HSV, and acyclovir triphosphate inhibits DNA polymerase.

127. *Nitric oxide:*
   (a) Is synthesised from L-arginine.
   (b) Is produced exclusively by endothelial cells.
   (c) Nitric oxide synthetases are cytokine-inducible.
   (d) Excess nitric oxide is implicated in essential hypertension.
   (e) It is the active moiety of glyceryl trinitrate.

128. *Antibiotics are appropriate for the infections:*
   (a) Cefotaxime: *Pseudomonas aeruginosa.*
   (b) Teicoplanin: *Haemophilus influenzae.*
   (c) Clarithromycin *Mycobacterium avium.*
   (d) Ceftriaxone: Enterococcal infections.
   (e) Clindamycin: *Staphylococcus aureus.*

129. *Neurofibromatosis type I (von Recklinghausen's disease):*
   (a) Is an autosomal dominant disorder.
   (b) Has an incidence of about 1:3500 in Western populations.
   (c) Almost all patients who inherit the neurofibromatosis type I gene have clinical features by the age of 5 years.
   (d) New mutations in this disorder are very rare.
   (e) About 90% of sporadic mutations in the NFI gene occur on the paternally inherited chromosome.

130. *Immunoglobulin deficiencies:*
   (a) Selective IgA deficiency is found in approximately 1: 3000 healthy subjects.
   (b) IgA deficiency may be transient, and can occur after the ingestion of penicillamine or gold.
   (c) IgG2 deficiency is more common in adults, and IgG3 deficiency in young children.
   (d) IgG sub-class deficiency in infancy and childhood is more common in boys than girls.
   (e) IgA deficiency may be associated with atopy, coeliac disease, SLE and Sjögren's syndrome.

131. *Sickle cell disease:*
    (a) Can be treated by bone marrow transplantation.
    (b) May be diagnosed antenatally.
    (c) Is a cause of proliferative retinopathy which frequently results in severe visual impairment.
    (d) May be complicated by megaloblastic erythropoiesis due to folate deficiency.
    (e) May be complicated by life-threatening pneumococcal septicaemia.

132. *Paget's disease:*
    (a) The male:female ratio is 3:1.
    (b) A combination of increased osteoblastic and osteoclastic activity occurs.
    (c) Osteocalcin has been shown to be a useful marker of response to treatment.
    (d) Calcitonin is the treatment of choice for Pagetic bone pain.
    (e) High-dose biphosphonate treatment is associated with defective mineralisation and fractures.

133. *Colony-stimulating factors (CSF):*
    (a) Are purified for clinical use from Buffy coats.
    (b) Are peptide hormones that bind to specific receptors on myeloid cells.
    (c) As a consequence of their long duration of action they are administered weekly.
    (d) Their co-administration with chemotherapeutic agents is not recommended.
    (e) Pulmonary oedema is a side-effect.

134. *Streptococcus pneumoniae:*
    (a) The vaccine immunizes against a surface antigen shared by pathogenic pneumococcal strains.
    (b) Penicillin resistance is rare in the western hemisphere.
    (c) Acapsular strains are more virulent.
    (d) Infections are increased in patients with HIV.
    (e) Neutrophilia is a poor prognostic sign in pneumococcal pneumonia.

135. *Multiple endocrine neoplasia type 2:*
    (a) Is caused by mutation of the *RET* proto-oncogene.
    (b) Is dominantly inherited.
    (c) In this condition, raised plasma catecholamines or calcitonin may indicate that the individual is affected.
    (d) Pancreatic islet adenomas affect about 80% of patients with this condition.
    (e) Genetic screening may yield ambiguous results and does not add to biochemical screening tests.

136. *Syndrome X as described by cardiologists:*
    (a) Is associated with insulin resistance.
    (b) Pro-insulin levels and C-peptide levels may be raised.
    (c) May be related to endothelial dysfunction in the cardiac microvasculature.
    (d) Is usually associated with single vessel coronary atheroma and a positive exercise test.
    (e) Is associated with impaired EDRF activity.

137. *The biology of interferons:*
    (a) Interferon-α has been used in the treatment of chronic active hepatitis B and C, hairy cell leukaemia, and multiple myeloma.
    (b) Most viruses and non-viral mitogens, such as phytohaemagglutinin and concanavalin-A mainly stimulate the production of interferon-γ by T lymphocytes.
    (c) Inteferons-α β and γ have a common cellular receptor.
    (d) Interferon-α is myelosuppressive and may cause hypotension, fever and infiltrative pulmonary disease when used therapeutically.
    (e) Interferon-γ may have a role in the therapy of relapsing-remitting multiple sclerosis.

138. *Cheese:*
     (a) There is an increased risk of infection with *E coli, Salmonella paratyphi,* and *Listeria monocytogenes* in patients who eat cheese made from unpasteurised milk.
     (b) In the EU, manufacturers are obliged to state on the retail label of their products that they were made from unpasteurised milk.
     (c) Haemolytic–uraemic syndrome may develop as a consequence of eating cheese made from unpasteurised cows' or goats' milk.
     (d) Vomiting which develops within a few hours of ingestion of a contaminated product is likely to be due to streptococcal enterotoxin.
     (e) Pregnant women and immunocompromised patients should be advised to avoid cheese made from unpasteurised milk.

139. *Familial hypercholesterolaemia:*
     (a) Is caused by mutations in the gene for the low density lipoprotein receptor.
     (b) Causes primary type IIa or IIb hyperlipidaemia.
     (c) In homozygous form may be associated with myocardial infarction in the second decade of life.
     (d) Treatment with inhibitors of the enzyme hydroxy methyl glutaryl CoA (HMGCoA) reductase may exacerbate the metabolic abnormality.
     (e) Is mimicked by mutations in the apolipoprotein B (apo B) gene causing familial defective apo B.

140. *Infection with HIV:*
     (a) HIV typically induces a granulomatous reaction in lymph nodes.
     (b) Activation of the transcription factor NF-kB inhibits HIV replication.
     (c) After primary infection HIV replication ceases and the virus enters a latent state.
     (d) CD8 is the main binding site for HIV on T cells.
     (e) HIV preferentially infects activated T cells.

141. *The human genome:*
   (a) Introns in genes contain only functionless DNA.
   (b) There are approximately 100 000 genes.
   (c) 1 centiMorgan is equivalent to a probability of recombination of 1% at meiosis.
   (d) Non-functional genes (pseudogenes) are rarely found.
   (e) Microsatellites (short tandem repeats) are useful polymorphic markers.

142. *Hyponatraemia (>120 mmol l^{-1} Na):*
   (a) Is commonly associated with over-hydration after surgery.
   (b) May be due to SIADH.
   (c) Is rarely associated with clouding of consciousness.
   (d) Should be corrected in most cases at a minimum rate of 10 mmol l^{-1} per 24 h.
   (e) May result in swelling of cells within the brain, with an initial rise in intracellular potassium.

143. *Hypocomplementaemic urticarial vasculitis:*
   (a) Is associated with auto-antibodies to C1q.
   (b) Is usually associated with positive anti-nuclear antibodies in most patients.
   (c) Is associated with chronically low levels of C4.
   (d) Rarely responds to therapy with dapsone or anti-malarials.
   (e) Is a cause of a mononeuritis multiplex.

144. *Proto-oncogenes may encode the following:*
   (a) Growth factors.
   (b) Growth factor receptors.
   (c) Transcription factors.
   (d) Protein kinases.
   (e) Complement proteins.

145. *Cryoglobulinaemia:*
   (a) Is a common cause of Raynaud's phenomenon.
   (b) May occur in SLE.
   (c) Is typically associated with very low C4 and C3 levels in plasma.
   (d) May suggest an underlying lymphoproliferative disorder.
   (e) May make cardiac surgery potentially hazardous.

146. *Gastric acid secretion:*
    (a) Is consistently increased in patients with duodenal ulceration.
    (b) Is inhibited by somatostatin produced by mucosal G-cells.
    (c) Is increased in asymptomatic *Helicobacter pylori* positive subjects.
    (d) Is stimulated by gastrin-releasing peptide.
    (e) Is reduced by Lanzoprazole therapy.

147. *The following are useful biochemical markers of alcohol abuse:*
    (a) Plasma aspartate transaminase.
    (b) Gammaglutamyl tranferase.
    (c) Plasma phosphate level.
    (d) Mitochondrial aspartate transaminase.
    (e) α-Glutathione S-transferase.

148. *Anti-oxidants:*
    (a) May inhibit atherogenesis by inhibiting the oxidative modification of low density lipoprotein particles by free radicals.
    (b) May reduce the carcinogenic potential of damaged nucleic acids.
    (c) Are present at high levels in red meat.
    (d) Include vitamins E, C, A and D.
    (e) Include the flavonoid group of compounds present at high levels in apples, onions and red wine.

149. *Insulin therapy:*
    (a) Human, pork and beef insulin are all equally immunogenic.
    (b) A preparation marked 'prb' implies that the drug was made biosynthetically in bacteria or yeast.
    (c) Insulatard (human or pork), and Humulin I/Zn preparations have an onset between 3 and 6 h after administration, and last up to 24 h.
    (d) Mixtard insulins exhibit 'biphasic' pharmacodynamics, and have an onset after 30 min, with peak efficacy betwen 1 and 12 h.
    (e) Multiple injection regimens including four or more injections per day have clearly been shown to improve glycaemic control and reduce long-term complications of diabetes.

150. *Pregnancy:*
   (a) In a normal woman, pregnancy is often associated with an elevated blood urea and albumin.
   (b) Is associated with higher than normal levels of many complement proteins.
   (c) Low-dose prednisolone is contraindicated for the treatment of rheumatic disorders.
   (d) Anti-phospholipid antibodies may result in spontaneous abortion.
   (e) Patients with SLE should be advised to avoid pregnancy if at all possible, as a post-delivery flare frequently occurs.

151. *Nephrotic syndrome:*
   (a) Hypertension is commonly associated with minimal change nephropathy.
   (b) Angiotensin converting enzyme inhibitors may reduce proteinuria by 50%.
   (c) Membranous nephropathy resolves spontaneously in up to 10% of patients.
   (d) Corticosteroids induce remission of membranous nephropathy in 90% of patients.
   (e) Minimal change nephropathy is associated with hepatitis B infection.

152. *Complications of infectious mononucleosis:*
   (a) Splenic rupture.
   (b) Myocarditis.
   (c) Polyneuritis.
   (d) Meningitis.
   (e) Glomerulonephritis.

153. *Cancer genetics:*
    (a) Hereditary non-polyposis colon cancer (HNPCC) is the commonest form of inherited colon cancer.
    (b) HNPCC families may also have cancers of the stomach, endometrium and ovary.
    (c) Mutations in the *BRCA1* gene are present in around 50% of families with inherited breast cancer, and are also responsible for many cases of inherited male breast cancer.
    (d) HNPCC individuals have mutations in MMR (mis-match repair) genes.
    (e) Mutations in MMR genes may result in a replication error phenotype.

154. *Growth hormone:*
    (a) Induces expression of insulin-like growth factor 1 in cardiac muscle tissue.
    (b) Deficiency results in impaired cardiac development with a reduction in myocardial mass.
    (c) May be administered in recombinant form to congenitally deficient subjects.
    (d) Is a potential target for drug abuse.
    (e) May have a future role in the treatment of cardiac failure.

155. *Genetic disorders:*
    (a) Lesch–Nyhan syndrome is an autosomal recessive disorder due to deficiency of the enzyme hypoxanthine guanine phosphoribosyl transferase.
    (b) Tay-Sachs disease is a G_{M2} gangliosidosis due to a genetic defect in hexosaminidase A.
    (c) The phenotype of patients with Hunter syndrome is less severe than that of Hurler syndrome.
    (d) Enzymopathies are almost always recessive.
    (e) Mortality in Z/Z genotype α_1-anti-trypsin deficient patients over the age of 60 is 6-fold higher in smokers.

Answers and
Explanatory Notes

1. (a) F.
   (b) T.
   (c) T.
   (d) F.
   (e) T.
   The major structural genes of HIV are: *Gag* which encodes for nucleocapsid core proteins such as p24, p9 and p17. *Pol* contains the genes for the major enzymes involved in HIV replication, namely reverse transcriptase, protease and integrase. *Env* is responsible for the outer envelope proteins gp120 and gp41 that are involved in entry of HIV into cells. HIV does contain a '*Rev*' gene but this has nothing to do with reverse transcriptase and is important in nuclear trafficking of HIV proteins. In addition there are *Tat*, *Nef*, *Vpr* and *Vpu* genes involved in regulation of various stages of the HIV life cycle. Inside the core of the HIV virus are two copies of the RNA genome. Newly formed HIV particles fuse with the T-cell membrane and then bud from the cell surface acquiring host proteins as infectious virus is released.

2. (a) F. This is the key difference between the classic genetic approach which required knowledge of the biochemical defect of a disorder in order to identify the mutant protein and gene. Positional cloning requires no such knowledge.
   (b) F. Susceptibility genes for breast cancer and Alzheimer's disease were identified by positional cloning.
   (c) T. The term 'reverse genetics' is not now generally used, however.
   (d) T.
   (e) T.

3. (a) T.
   (b) T.
   (c) F.

(d) F.
(e) F.
Deficiency of classical complement components C1q, C2 and C4 are associated with the development of lupus. 28 out of the 30 or so C1q deficient patients described had SLE, while C2 deficiency confers a 33% risk of developing the disease. This is thought to be due to impairment of the processing of immune complexes. There is also an acquired reduction in the complement receptor type 1 (CR1), a glycoprotein present on the surface of red cells in primates, in lupus patients. This receptor is involved in the carriage of immune complexes in the circulation, and while the mechanism of its loss in the disease is not fully understood, it may be related to proteolytic loss of part of a receptor from the red cell surface, consequent upon immune complex removal in the liver and spleen. While deficiency of terminal pathway complement components (which comprise the membrane attack complex) is associated with increased susceptibility to Neisserial disease, there is epidemiological evidence that the disease is less severe in affected patients. This may be because there is a blunting of the inflammatory response to infection in the absence of complement, with a reduction in complement mediated cell lysis and endotoxin release.

C1 inhibitor deficiency does predispose to hereditary angiooedema, but the patients are heterozygotes. Homozygous deficiency is not described. C1 inhibitor levels in affected heterozygous patients are usually somewhat less than the expected 50%, due to accelerated catabolism of the product of the normal allele.

It is useful to monitor complement levels in patients with SLE, but of no value in microscopic polyangiitis, Wegener's, or Churg–Strauss Syndrome, in which systemic complement consumption is not a major feature.

4. (a) T.
   (b) F.
   (c) T.
   (d) F.
   (e) T.
Hepatitis A is an RNA picornavirus while hepatitis C is a positive-stranded RNA virus of 9379 nucleotides classified within the Flaviviridae. Chronic infection develops in up to 50% of those infected with hepatitis C and interferon-α is a

useful treatment although relapse is usual on stopping treatment. Hepatitis D virus (delta agent) is a defective RNA virus found only in the presence of active hepatitis B and is usually seen in drug-abusers or multiply-transfused patients. Hepatitis E is an RNA virus transmitted by the faeco-oral route. It is an epidemic form of hepatitis found in Asia, the Indian sub-continent and North Africa. The infection is acute and usually self-limiting, however it is particularly severe in pregnant women with up to 40% mortality. The complications of hepatitis C infection include chronic hepatitis and cirrhosis and occasionally systemic vasculitis and cryoglobulinaemia.

5. (a) T.
    (b) F.
    (c) T.
    (d) T.
    (e) F.
    The human herpes viruses identified to date are: HSV 1 and 2, VZV, EBV, CMV, HHV6, HHV7 and HHV8. HHV6 causes roseola infantum (exanthum subitum), a mononucleosis-like illness in adults and pneumonitis in severely immunocompromised hosts. HHV7 is still looking for a disease and HHV8 has recently been detected in KS lesions from all groups of patients. B virus is a simian herpes virus that has caused fatal disease in humans following laboratory exposure to monkeys, it will respond to acyclovir. Acyclovir is phosphorylated by a herpes virus-encoded thymidine kinase and then further phosphorylated to the active triphosphate form by host kinases. Foscarnet is an analogue of pyrophosphate and inhibits herpes viral replication by irreversibly binding to the pyrophosphate acceptor site on DNA polymerase.

6. (a) T. Heterozygosity is when two alleles of a marker are seen, for example on a southern blot or by PCR amplification and gel electrophoresis. Loss of heterozygosity is when two alleles are present on analysis of peripheral blood lymphocyte DNA but only one allele is seen on analysis of tumour DNA. This suggests that one copy has been lost from tumour DNA implying a chromosomal deletion. This may contribute to tumorigenesis if an adjacent gene, also deleted, is a tumour suppressor gene.
    (b) F. Lyonisation or random X-chromosome inactivation is the process of inactivation of a whole X-chromosome in female

somatic cells. In a normal tissue either the paternal or maternal X-chromosome is inactivated at random, whereas in a mono-clonal tumour either the paternal or maternal X-chromosome is always inactivated. This allows assignment of monoclonality in females but **not** in males.

(c) F. In inherited retinoblastoma one mutation is somatic and the other is germline.

(d) F. In the multi-step path to tumour formation, oncogene activation and tumour suppressor gene inactivation may both play a part.

(e) T. Two notable examples are the Rb gene and the p53 gene.

7. (a) F.
   (b) T.
   (c) F.
   (d) T.
   (e) F.

Fas is a 43 kDa glycoprotein molecule involved in inducing apoptosis in lymphocytes, but both B and T cells are involved. Although up to 60% of lupus patients do have measurable levels of soluble Fas protein in their serum, the levels of Fas protein on the surface of freshly isolated peripheral B cells, and of CD4- and CD8-positive T lymphocytes from patients with SLE were also found to be higher than in normal controls.

Transcription of the *Fas* gene is defective in MRL/lpr lupus-prone mice, but this results in **defective** apoptosis. Longer survival of apoptosis-resistant autoreactive lymphocytes may be involved in the development of autoimmunity, or it may be the case that such cells which are not processed by the normal apoptotic pathway, present autoantigens in an inappropriate manner to the immune system. B cell hyperactivity, largely as a consequence of T-cell driven help are features both of human SLE and the MRL/IPR murine lupus model.

8. (a) T.
   (b) T.
   (c) F.
   (d) F.
   (e) T.

In the initial incubation period in the hepatocyte the exo-erythrocytic schizonts are found prior to direct invasion of erythrocytes. Haemoglobin S heterozygotes (AS) are protected against the lethal complications of malaria with *P. falciparum* growing poorly in red cells containing HbS. The incubation time is 7–10 days for falciparum malaria and longer for other species and the onset may be insidious. Complications of falciparum malaria include cerebral malaria, acute renal failure, hepatic failure, severe diarrhoea and vomiting and Blackwater fever, the result of rapid intravascular haemolysis more common in those who have taken anti-malarials infrequently and those with G-6-PD deficiency. Nephrotic syndrome is a complication of *P. malariae*.

9. (a) T.
   (b) F.
   (c) T.
   (d) T.
   (e) F.
   Bartonella (Rochalimea) hensulae and *B. quintana* have been identified as the cause of cat scratch disease. In AIDS patients these organisms are responsible for bacilliary angiomatosis, pyrexia of unknown origin and peliosis hepatitis. Bacilliary angiomatosis presents with multiple vascular skin lesions that resemble Kaposi sarcomata. Fluconazole and ketoconazole have no useful activity against *Aspergillus* spp. Itraconazole does exhibit anti-aspergillus activity and may be useful for maintenance therapy but amphotericin B remains the treatment of choice for active disease.
   Progressive multifocal leukoencephalopathy is due to infection of the brain with a number of polyoma viruses. These are DNA viruses including JC, BK and SV40.
   Cryptosporidium parvae is one of the most commonly identified causes of diarrhoea in AIDS. Cryptosporidia line the mucosa of both the small and large bowel; they do not disrupt the gut mucosal integrity and the mechanism of diarrhoea is incompletely understood. CMV pneumonitis is a major cause of death in transplant recipients but much less common in the context of HIV.

10. (a) T. Trinucleotide repeats are a type of microsatellite and are hypervariable, i.e highly polymorphic.
    (b) F. In Huntington's chorea the trinucleotide repeat is expanded not contracted.
    (c) T. Anticipation is the appearance of a disease at progressively

earlier age in successive generations and is due to progressive expansion of the repeat element.

(d) F. Some trinucleotide repeat elements are within the coding sequence of functional proteins, for example, Huntington's disease, Kennedy disease, and spinocerebellar ataxia type I.

(e) T. The fragile X syndrome was the first example of this type.

11. (a) T.
    (b) T.
    (c) T.
    (d) F.
    (e) T.

Perinuclear anti-neutrophil cytoplasmic antibodies are found in the serum of some patients with Crohn's disease. There is an association in this patient group with a rare allele (R241) of the ICAM-1 gene, and there is evidence that the ANCA positive Crohn's disease patients have a clinical phenotype which overlaps somewhat with that of ulcerative colitis. These patients frequently have symptoms of left-sided colitis, and may have histological features which resemble those of UC. An anti-erythrocyte antibody derived from the VH3-15 gene (AEA15) has been shown to be elevated in serum from Crohn's disease patients, and to occur at lower levels in UC patients and those with *Campylobacter* infection. It is not presently clear whether this autoantibody has any pathogenic role.

There are associations with HLA class II (DR and DQ) genes, and a specific TNF microsatellite haplotype in 25% of patients. This haplotype defines a subset of Crohn's patients who produce high levels of TNF in response to *in vitro* leukocyte activation. There is no association with the HLA class III (complement) genes which are also encoded on chromosome 6.

Anti-TNF monoclonal antibodies have been shown in a small study to be very effective, producing prolonged disease amelioration in some patients with Crohn's disease.

12. (a) T.
    (b) T.
    (c) F.
    (d) T.
    (e) T.

Metronidazole is used in acute amoebic dysentry, amoebic abscesses and also trichomonas vaginalis. Diloxanide is the treatment of choice in chronic intestinal amoebiasis whilst sodium stibogluconate is the treatment of choice for visceral leishmaniasis. Most cases of toxoplasmosis are self-limiting and do not require specific treatment. However, treatment is required in the immunosuppressed and those with eye involvement and a combination of sulphonamide and pyrimethamine is the treatment of choice. Tetracyclines are an alternative. Nebulised and intravenous pentamidine is effective against pneumocystis although co-trimoxazole is the agent of choice.

13. (a) T.
    (b) F.
    (c) F.
    (d) T.
    (e) F.
    Cyclospora is a coccidian parasite that has been described as a cause of diarrhoea in travellers to central Asia and in patients with HIV. *Clostridium difficile* occasionally causes pseudomem-branous colitis without antibiotic exposure particularly in the immunocompromised host. *Giardia lamblia* is one parasite that does not cause eosinophilia. Enterohaemorrhagic *E. coli* (particularly strain 0157) are one of the main precipitants of the haemolytic uraemic syndrome presenting with renal failure, thrombocytopenia and microangiopathic haemolytic anaemia. *Bacillus cereus* produces a heat-stable enterotoxin that causes acute food poisoning within hours of ingestion.

14. (a) F. X-linked dominant traits follow Mendelian inheritance (e.g. X-linked hypophosphataemia).
    (b) T. Leprosy and tuberculosis in the past have been considered as genetic disorders.
    (c) T, because all mitochondrial DNA is inherited from the mother.
    (d) T. Non-Mendelian inheritance may result in false-negative linkage results.
    (e) T. Uniparental isodisomy has occurred if a child inherits both copies of a chromosome from one parent. This contravenes the rules of Mendelian inheritance.

15. (a) F.
    (b) T.
    (c) T.

(d) F.
(e) F.

Nitric oxide is a ubiquitous vasodilator. It is synonymous with endothelium-derived relaxing factor (EDRF). It is generated from its substrate L-arginine by NO synthase of which there are a number of types: inducible NO synthase (iNOS), neuronal nitric oxide synthase (nNOS), and endothelial nitric oxide synthase. The latter is activated by receptor G-protein coupling in response to a wide range of stimuli including circulating hormones such as bradykinin, and neurotransmitters such as acetylcholine and substance P. There is increasing contemporary interest in the role of longitudinal shear stress in the generation of nitric oxide production.

Nitric oxide prevents platelet aggregation and adhesion to the vessel wall, and in the heart it increases diastolic compliance and reduces the duration of contraction. It has little effect on systolic contraction, and overall favours filling in diastole.

Nitric oxide activity is impaired by endothelial dysfunction, and there is increasing interest in the role of this mediator in the process of atherogenesis. A number of mechanisms have been suggested, and it is possible that NO may be anti-atherogenic in that it scavenges oxygen free radicals, and can prevent the attraction of inflammatory cells into atheromatous lesions. Its capacity to increase cyclic GMP, will also have an anti-proliferative effect.

16. (a) T.
    (b) F.
    (c) T.
    (d) T.
    (e) F.

Antihelminthics are reasonably effective in the treatment of threadworm infections, provided that treatment is combined with appropriate hygiene measures and that all members of the family are treated. The treatment of choice is mebendazole in those over 2 years of age, given as a single dose. Niclosamide and praziquantel are the most effective taenicides while the treatment of strongyloidiasis is thiabendazole. Other important infections in this group include hydatid disease for which the treatment involves albendazole and surgery as required. The treatment of hookworm infection requires mebendazole or pyrantel to remove the worm and in addition, treatment to correct the anaemia associated with the disease. Schistosomiasis of all types is effectively treated with praziquantel whilst diethylcarbamazine is the drug of choice in filarial infections. Finally, treatment of strongyloidiasis is a course of thiabendazole or alternatively albendazole.

17. (a) F.
    (b) F.
    (c) F.
    (d) T.
    (e) F.
    Lipopolysaccharide (endotoxin, LPS) is a glucosamine-based phospholipid that is found in the outer leaflet of all Gram-negative bacteria. LPS is responsible for many of the pathophysiological changes leading to septic shock in patients with Gram-negative infection. Auramine staining is used for TB and other acid-fast organisms, pneumocystis can be detected with giemsa and silver stains or by immunofluorescent antibody techniques. *Listeria monocytogenes* is a Gram-positive rod. The coagulase enzyme of *S. aureus* interacts with the D fragment of fibrinogen. The coagulase test is used to distinguish *S. aureus* from other Staphylococci and is therefore of prime importance in the rapid evaluation of the pathological significance of staphylococcal isolates. Visualising *Cryptosporidium parvae* requires specific staining techniques, since it is an acid-fast organism and so can be detected with modified Ziehl–Nielsson or auramine stains.

18. (a) F. In the past, accumulation of *aluminium* not magnesium has been debated in Alzheimer's pathogenesis.
    (b) T.
    (c) F. Familial Alzheimer's with early onset frequently has dominant inheritance.
    (d) T. In monogenic Alzheimer's DNA sequence analysis may indicate disease predisposition.
    (e) T. Possibly because of the extra copy of the gene for serum amyloid protein on chromosome 21.

19. (a) T.
    (b) T.
    (c) T.
    (d) T.
    (e) F.

Anti–neutrophil cytoplasmic antibodies are useful in diagnosis and monitoring of systemic vasculitis. Using the standard immuno-fluorescence method a positive ANCA may be reported in patients with SLE who have high titre anti-nuclear antibodies. The specific antibodies themselves do not occur in lupus, however, and this is a 'false positive'. Anti-proteinase 3 is associated with Wegener's, and anti-myeloperoxidase antibodies occur in microscopic polyangitis. Disease severity, as measured by the number of organ systems involved, is not generally related to initial ANCA level. In many patients a rise in ANCA may predict a relapse in vasculitis.

20. (a) F.
    (b) T.
    (c) T.
    (d) F.
    (e) F.

Lyme disease was first described in 1982 in Lyme, Connecticut and the causative organism subsequently identified as *Borellia burgdorferi*. The organism is spread by the *Ixodes* tick with deer as the animal source. The tick bite results in a characteristic rash, erythema chronicum migrans. About 15% of patients develop neurological disease which may include cranial nerve palsies, lymphocytic meningitis, encephalitis and polyneuritis. Cardiac involvement is seen in 8% with an increase in P–R interval the commonest change and peri- or pancarditis, cardiomegaly and AV block also described. Joint symptoms are seen in up to 80% of patients and may appear months after the initial symptoms; a chronic arthritis is seen in approximately 10% of patients. Antibiotic treatment is of benefit if given early; penicillin, cephalosporins and tetracyclines are all effective.

21. (a) F.
    (b) F.
    (c) T.
    (d) F.
    (e) T.

Notification is the responsibility of the physician looking after the infected patient. Notification is an obligation under law and failure to notify is an offence. Sexually transmitted diseases and HIV are specifically not notifiable diseases as this would be counterproductive in identifying and treating infected indivi-duals. This is the current list of notifiable diseases in the UK:

Anthrax	Marburg disease	Relapsing fever
Cholera	Measles	Scarlet fever
Diphtheria	Meningitis (acute)	Smallpox
Dysentery	Ophthalmia	Tetanus
Encephalitis (acute)	neonatorum	Tuberculosis
Food poisoning	Plague	Typhoid fever
Infective jaundice	Polio	Typhus
Lassa fever	Paratyphoid fever	Viral haemolytic fevers
Leprosy	Rabies (acquired	Whooping cough
Leptospirosis	in UK)	Yellow fever
Malaria		

22. (a) F. Theoretically only one copy of the target sequence is required.
(b) F. Double-stranded product results, although asymmetric PCR with production of single-stranded product is possible.
(c) T. Diagnostic techniques of this type are presently only available in specialist centres, although they are increasing in availability throughout the UK.
(d) T.
(e) F. Knowledge of the DNA sequence is needed to design appropriate primers.

23. (a) T.
(b) F.
(c) T.
(d) F.
(e) T.
Xenoreactive antibodies are present in the serum of the potential human recipient. The main target antigen is a galactose-containing disaccharide. Hyperacute rejection is mediated by antibodies directed against this and other epitopes, which fix complement. Cells are not involved in the acute rejection process. This can be modified by genetic modification of the donor complement control proteins DAF and CD59, and genes for these human proteins have been introduced into the pig by transgenic methods. Recent studies suggest that a further useful strategy may be the enzymatic remodelling of this disaccharide antigen to resemble the blood group H antigen.

24. (a) T.
    (b) T.
    (c) F.
    (d) F.
    (e) T.

In order to prevent the clotting of blood in the extra-corporeal circulation 7500–15 000 units of heparin are generally administered to patients undergoing plasma exchange. The technique is of value in the treatment of various auto-immune disorders, including anti-GBM disease, rapidly progressive proliferative nephritis due to ANCA-positive vasculitides, thrombotic thrombocytopoenic purpura and both Guillain-Barré syndrome and chronic demyelinating polyneuropathies. It is used by a number of centres for the treatment of patients with acute lupus nephritis, though its value in the mangement of this condition remains to be conclusively proven. It is not used in the long-term management of SLE.

Plasma exchange is particularly effective for removing immunoglobulins and immune complexes from the intravascular comaprtment, and is therefore particularly effective in patients with hyperviscosity due to Waldenstrom's macroglobulinaemia or essential mixed cryoglobulinaemia. Both a fall in platelet count and haemoglobin may result from the procedure.

25. (a) F.
    (b) F.
    (c) F.
    (d) F.
    (e) F.

Ninety percent of renal blood flow is distributed to the cortex. NSAIDs render the kidney susceptible to the effects of endogenous vasoconstrictors, and therefore reduce renal blood flow. Care is therefore needed in the administration of these medications in patients with chronic renal impairment.

In a normal subject renal blood flow is tightly autoregulated over a range of systolic blood pressure from 75–175 mmHg. ACE *inhibitors* cause vasodilatation and this may be harmful in the presence of renovascular disease and significant renal artery stenosis, as in this situation effective filtration is largely maintained by constriction of the efferent vessels.

Urea clearance may underestimate GFR. Up to 50% urea may be reabsorbed, explaining why there is a relatively greater rise in urea than in creatinine in volume-depletion. Urea production is also variable, and may be low, for example in chronic liver disease.

26. (a) T.
    (b) F.
    (c) T.
    (d) F.
    (e) T.

A wide range of rheumatic syndromes have been described in association with HIV infection:

1. Septic arthritis and osteomyelitis: opportunistic infection in AIDS.
2. Culture negative disease resembling spondyloarthropathies: Reiter's syndrome; psoriatic type arthritis; undifferentiated spondyloarthropathies with enthesopathy and dactylitis.
3. Arthralgia syndromes.
4. Sjögren's syndrome (diffuse infiltrative lymphocytosis).
5. Polymyositis.
6. Miscellaneous vasculitides.

In any patient with HIV presenting with joint pain and swelling there should be a low threshold for joint aspiration to exclude a septic arthritis.

27. (a) T.
    (b) T.
    (c) F.
    (d) T.
    (e) F.

Corticosteroid therapy reduces cranial nerve damage in childhood meningitis and TB meningitis. The use of steroids in other forms of meningitis has not been validated. Several large trials, and recent meta-analyses, have shown that steroids do not improve mortality in septic shock and increase the rate of secondary infections. An exception to this is the toxaemic presentation of enteric fever where steroids improve outcome. Steroid use in cerebral malaria has also been shown to be ineffective and probably detrimental.

28. (a) F.
    (b) F.
    (c) F.
    (d) T.
    (e) F.
    Thrombolysis is potentially hazardous and the risk to the patient must be carefully balanced against possible benefits. The treatment is absolutely contraindicated in the first 18 weeks of pregnancy, intracranial aneurysm or tumour, aortic dissection, head injury, a stroke within the last two months, active gastro-intestinal haemorrhage and severe thrombocytopoenia. Diabetic proliferative retinopathy is a relative contraindication. Pupillary dilation with tropicamide or phenylephrine is recommended. Caution is obviously necessary in a hypertensive patient, cancer patients, after an organ biopsy, and around the time of parturition, and in patients with a previous, but no recent history of peptic ulcer disease. Allergic reactions to streptokinase, in particular, are not uncommon, and cases of later immune complex-mediated reactions have been reported in patients previously sensitised by streptococcal infection. The latter is obviously very common, and cannot be regarded as a contra-indication to thrombolysis, though it may be expedient to consider TPA or another agent rather than streptokinase in this situation.

29. (a) F. Gilbert's syndrome is an entirely benign and clinically inconsequential entity in adults.
    (b) T. The enzyme defect is in UDPGT.
    (c) T. Gilbert's syndrome has recently been shown to be due to UDPGT promoter defects whilst Crigler–Najjar disease is due to structural mutations in the gene encoding the enzyme.
    (d) F. It is characterised by **unconjugated** hyperbilirubinaemia.
    (e) F. Serum bilirubin concentration typically increases after food in Gilbert's syndrome.

30. (a) T.
    (b) F.
    (c) F.
    (d) F.
    (e) T.
    Measles, mumps, rubella, yellow fever and polio are all live vaccines while whooping cough, diphtheria, tetanus, typhoid,

cholera and hepatitis B are killed vaccines. Live vaccines are generally contraindicated in the immunosuppressed and pregnant women.

Recommended routine immunisation schedules are as follows:

Diptheria/tetanus/pertussis/polio/haemophilus influenzae type B

1st dose	2 months
2nd dose	3 months
3rd dose	6 months
Booster	4–5 years
Booster	15–18 years

Measles/mumps/rubella	12–18 months
Rubella	10–14 years for girls only if not had MMR
BCG	10–14 years

31. (a) F.
    (b) T.
    (c) F.
    (d) F.
    (e) T.
    All non-steroidal anti-inflammatory drugs (NSAIDS) are cyclooxygenase (COX) enzyme inhibitors which reduce the synthesis of prostaglandins. When taken at low doses NSAIDS act mainly as analgesics, whilst at higher doses they also reduce inflammation. Physiologically prostaglandins act to protect the gastric mucosa and to help maintain renal blood flow. Hence inhibition of their function results in the unwanted effects of gastrointestinal ulceration and renal toxicity. Two isoforms of cyclooxygenase have been described COX-1 and COX-2. COX-1 is thought to be the isoform predominantly associated with synthesis of prostaglandins for protection of the gastric mucosa. COX-2 is an inducible isoform and is predominantly involved in the inflammatory response. Considerable research effort is now focused on the development of drugs that inhibit COX-2 specifically, so as to achieve the anti-inflammatory effects of NSAIDS without the gastrointestinal toxicity. Two such compounds are nabumetone, a pro-drug whose active derivative only weakly inhibits COX-1, and etodolac which has similar properties. Provisional studies suggest that these drugs may have reduced gastrointestinal side-effects without losing anti-inflammatory efficacy.

32. (a) F.
    (b) F.
    (c) F.
    (d) T.
    (e) F.

At the current time the median period to the development of AIDS is 8–10 years. Although mucocutaneous candidiasis occurs in most patients with AIDS candidaemia is very rare unless the patient is also neutropenic. In immunocompromised patients reactivation of toxoplasmosis causes brain abscesses and less commonly myocarditis or pneumonia. Choroidoretinitis due to toxoplasmosis is almost exclusively confined to congenital acquisition of infection. TB and cryptococcus are the most frequent opportunistic infections in African patients whilst PCP is relatively uncommon. Cryptococcosis is more common in Africa and S. E. Asia than Europe or the USA. In patients with HIV infection the most common cause of thrombocytopaenia is ITP, presumably antibody-mediated.

33. (a) T.
    (b) T.
    (c) F.
    (d) T.
    (e) F.

The Delta trial compared AZT (zidovudine) alone with AZT +DDI (didanosine) and AZT + DDC (zalcitidine) in patients with symptomatic HIV infection or AIDS. At 24 months follow-up there was a significant reduction in progression to AIDS and improved survival in patients receiving combination treatment rather than monotherapy. In vitro AZT inhibits HTLV-1 as well as HIV-1 and HIV-2 and has been used in combination with interferon-α to treat HTLV-1-associated lymphoma. Pancreatitis is the most serious side-effect of DDI; peripheral neuropathy is a limiting factor in patients receiving DDC. Perinatal transmission of HIV is reduced by 50% with maternal zidovudine therapy during the last trimester of pregnancy. HIV resistance to zidovudine (and other reverse transcriptase inhibitors) is mediated by mutations in the Pol gene encoding for the reverse transcriptase enzyme.

34. (a) T.
    (b) F. Mitochondrial DNA is **all** maternally inherited.

(c) T. Heteroplasmy means that different cells may have a varying proportion of mutated mitochondrial genomes. This might be part of the explanation of why (e) is true.

(d) T.

(e) T. The relationship between phenotype and genotypic abnormalities is poorly understood at present.

35. (a) F. The correction of defects in human germ cells is deemed to be unethical; all protocols to date have used somatic cells.

(b) T. Increased ADA activity, an increase in T cell numbers, an improvement in many immune functions and a decreased number of infectious illnesses have been demonstrated in this immunodeficiency disease after gene therapy.

(c) F. Retroviral vectors have been used for gene therapy. The potentially harmful retroviral genes for reverse transcriptase and other retroviral components are removed prior to their use.

(d) F. Gene therapy may be considered in patients who have null alleles in both disease genes. These patients will have not 'seen' the deficient protein in postnatal life and may therefore have the capacity to mount an immune response against the replaced protein.

(e) F. Although many patients with cystic fibrosis and all patients with sickle cell disease are true homozygotes, this does not seem to have a major impact on the success or failure of gene therapy.

36. (a) F.

(b) T.

(c) T.

(d) T.

(e) T.

CR1 is found on red blood cells in primates, but also on leukocytes, and glomerular epithelial cells. The receptor is clustered on erythrocytes, and it is these cells which are important in the safe carriage of immune complexes in the circulation. CR1 is a co-factor for factor I-mediated catabolism of C3, and sCR1 has been used in a number of experimental models to modify inflammatory processes in which complement is thought to be critical. It was first shown to be effective in this role in a rabbit model of reperfusion-induced myocardial ischaemia.

37. (a) T.
    (b) T.
    (c) T.
    (d) T.
    (e) F.

Acute intermittent porphyria affects females more commonly than males. It is unusual for patients to present in childhood or infancy, and the disease normally presents in the third decade. Abdominal symptoms are common, and may be manifest as constipation, diarrhoea, vomiting or abdominal pain. Two-thirds of patients develop a peripheral neuropathy, which is primarily motor, and affects the upper extremeties more than the lower limbs. Sensory symptoms may also occur, and occasionally the cranial nerves may be affected.

Grand mal epilepsy is reported in one fifth to one quarter of patients, and psychiatric symptoms, including psychosis and depression are reported in 50% of cases. The other clinical features which may be manifest during an acute attack include, tachycardia, heart failure, proteinuria, uraemia, leukocytosis and fever. Increased ADH secretion may result in hyponatraemia.

AIP results in chronically raised levels of porphobilinogen and δ-aminolaevulinic acid in the urine, and levels may rise further with an acute attack. Classically the diagnosis may be confirmed by detection of porphobilinogen using Ehrlich's aldehyde reagent. This turns pink, and is insoluble in chloroform/butanol, in contrast to urobilinogen, which is readily soluble (though also turns pink). Urine may turn orange/brown on standing.

Attacks may be precipitated by pregnancy, menstruation, intercurrent infection and alcohol. In young women dieting may also be a factor. Drugs are the commonest precipitants, notably barbiturates, the oral contraceptive pill and sulphonamides.

38. (a) T.
    (b) T.
    (c) F.
    (d) T.
    (e) T.

Amyloidosis is a disorder of protein-processing characterised by the extracellular deposition of amyloid fibrils, which have distinct ultrastructural properties. It is the accumulation of these fibrils in the tissues which causes organ failure. Mutations of the plasma protein transthyretin are the commonest cause of familial amyloid polyneuropathy, which is the most common type of hereditary amyloidosis. Mutations of apo-lipoprotein A1 (Apo-A1) can also cause amyloid. Mutations of arg56 and arg60 are known to be amyloidogenic, in particular. The arg56 variant may cause neuropathic and non-neuropathic amyloid, whilst apo-A1 arg60 is associated with non-neuropathic autosomal dominant amyloidosis.

Amyloid deposition in the presence of a persistent acute phase response may indeed regress with appropriate therapy. The best example of amyloid regression is in juvenile inflammatory arthritis.

Serum amyloid P component (SAP) scans are a sensitive and specific way of diagnosis and monitoring patients with systemic amyloidosis.

39. (a) T.
    (b) F.
    (c) T.
    (d) T.
    (e) T.

Six diseases of animals and four of humans as a result of prions have been described. These disorders are transmissible in some cases but may also be caused by mutations in the prion protein, which is encoded by a chromosomal gene. These disorders have a long incubation period and commonly cause a slowly progressive dementia with a characteristic spongiform encephalopathy. Most cases of Gerstmann–Sträussler–Scheinker (GSS) disease are familial and exhibit an autosomal dominant pattern of inheritance with almost complete penetrance. On clinical grounds it is said that GSS can be distinguished from Creutzfeld–Jakob disease (CJD) by the prominence of ataxia in GSS and the prominence of dementia with myoclonus in CJD. The problem of transmission to man of prion diseases remains a subject of intense debate. However, accidental transfer of CJD has been reported following corneal transplantation, contaminated EEG electrodes, contaminated instruments and via growth hormone isolated from cadaveric pituitary glands.

40. (a) F.
    (b) T.
    (c) F.
    (d) T.
    (e) T.
    The term scleroderma includes a variety of disorders including localised scleroderma (morphea), diffuse cutaneous scleroderma (systemic sclerosis) and CREST syndrome. Antibodies to Sclero-derma-70 (Scl-70) are present in approximately 25% of patients and are directed against a topoisomerase-1 which is a DNA charging enzyme. Anti-endothelial cell antibodies are distinct from the conventional connective tissue disease associated autoantibodies, including anti-dsDNA, and may activate endothelial cells and induce adhesion molecule expression. These antibodies have been described in a number of connective tissue diseases including scleroderma, systemic lupus erythematosus and Kawaski's disease. Although immunosuppressive drugs are probaly indicated early in the diffuse form of scleroderma there is no evidence that they significantly retard disease expression. Raynaud's phenomenon may precede scleroderma by 30 years and hypertension is commonly seen in these patients and may be resistant to treatment.

41. (a) T.
    (b) T.
    (c) T.
    (d) T.
    (e) F.
    There are five species of schistosomes that cause the majority of human infection. *S. haematobium* (terminal spine), *S. mansoni* (lateral spine), *S. japonicum* (small lateral spine), *S. intercalatum* (terminal spine) and *S. mekongi* (small lateral spine). *S. haematobium* preferentially infects the vesical venous plexus with the other species in the portal tract. *S. haematobium* eggs are often found on rectal biopsy but they are almost always dead. Katayama fever is an acute illness characterised by fever, myalgia, pulmonary infiltrates and eosinophilia. Katayama fever is due to the host response at the onset of egg production by the adult worms. The characteristic histological response to the eggs is a granulomatous reaction and in the liver this eventually leads to cirrhosis. Widespread dissemination of the eggs can occur and paraplegia due to spinal cord involvement is well recognised. The therapy of choice is praziquantel.

42. (a) T. Genomic imprinting is used to describe the situation in which only the paternal *or* maternal gene is expressed. One proposed mechanism for this is by methylation of the DNA in the 'silent' or 'imprinted' gene or chromosome segment.
(b) F. Genomic imprinting was first discovered in mice.
(c) T. The imprinting or suppression of maternal genes on chromosome 15q11 means that these genes are not expressed. All recorded cases of Prader–Willi syndrome arise on the paternally inherited chromosome 15. Deletions in the same region of the maternal chromosome 15 lead to Angelman syndrome.
(d) F. Genomic imprinting is systematic unlike Lyonisation (see question 6 above) which is random.
(e) F. Genomic imprinting is an autosomal phenomenon; sex-linked muscular dystrophies are X-linked genetic disorders.

43. (a) F.
    (b) F.
    (c) T.
    (d) F.
    (e) T.
Drug-induced abnormalities in liver function tests generally resolve within a few weeks of stopping therapy. Persistent abnormalities may require further investigation. A combined hepatitic and cholestatic picture may occur with tricyclics, anti-TB drugs (ethambutol, pyrizinamide and ethambutol), erythromycin, nitrofurantoin, fusidic acid, ampicilin, and phenothiazines such as chlorpromazine. Indocid and certain other NSAIDs can also produce this picture, as well as benzodiazepines, and both oestrogens and androgen derivatives.

Inhalational anaesthetics typically give a hepatitic picture, as do methyldopa, isoniazid and certain MAO inhibitors. Tetracycline may be directly toxic to the liver and cause steatosis, and methotrexate may be associated with fatty infiltration portal fibrosis or cirrhosis. With the prolonged use of the drug at low dose in psoriasis or RA, some physicians recommend liver biopsy at 12–18-month intervals, as biochemical liver function tests are not necessarily a good guide to toxicity.

44. (a) F.
    (b) F.
    (c) T.

(d) T.
(e) T.
There is considerable variation in CD4/CD8 ratios in normal subjects. In one series of 486 healthy blood donors, the ratio varied between 0.39 and 7.43. This appears to be partly genetically controlled, and to remain relatively constant within any one individual. The ratio is generally lower in males than females, attributable mainly to a lower number of CD4 positive cells. The ratio increases with age, and is useful in monitoring patients infected with HIV, in whom the ratio shows a decline with the onset of symptomatic AIDS.

The ratio is generally low in patients with acute viral infections, allograft rejection, haemophilia, and host versus graft disease.

45. (a) T.
    (b) F.
    (c) T.
    (d) T.
    (e) F.
Infection with parvovirus B19 may result in a variety of clinical manifestations including erythema infectiosum (fifth disease, slapped cheek syndrome), acute arthritis, hydrops fetalis, transient aplastic crisis, and rarely a vasculitis, peripheral neuropathy, nephritis and myocarditis. Vasculitis has also been described in association with hepatitis B, hepatitis C and HIV infection. The C reactive protein is often a useful marker of vasculitic disease activity. However it may also be increased by co-existent infection. Anti-neutrophil cytoplasmic antibodies (ANCA) were first described in 1982 and are divided on the basis of their staining pattern into cANCA (cytoplasmic) and pANCA (perinuclear). Approximately 80% of patients with active Wegener's granulomatosis have cANCA antibodies whilst pANCA is found in 50% of patients with microscopic polyarteritis. The pANCA is less specific and less sensitive than cANCA and is found in polyarteritis nodosa, rheumatoid vasculitis, Kawasaki's syndrome and idiopathic segmental necrotising glomerulonephritis.

Vasculitis may affect all sizes of vessels, e.g. Giant cell arteritis and Takayasu's arteritis (large arteries); Kawasaki's syndrome and polyarteritis nodosa (medium arteries); Henoch–Schönlein purpura and polyangiitis (small vessels).

46. (a) F.
    (b) F.
    (c) T.
    (d) F.
    (e) T.
Hepatitis E is mainly transmitted by the fecal/oral route. The delta agent (hepatitis D) is a defective RNA virus that requires active hepatitis B viral replication in order to produce complete viral particles that utilise hepatitis B surface antigen to form the viral envelope. Approximately 50% of patients with hepatitis C will develop chronic infection and at least 70% of these will progress to cirrhosis. Between 40 and 60% of patients with chronic hepatitis B infection will respond to interferon-α. Hepatitis A, C, D and E are RNA viruses while hepatitis B has a double stranded DNA genome.

47. (a) T.
    (b) T.
    (c) T.
    (d) F.
    (e) F.
In tuberculoid leprosy there is a strong cell-mediated immune response characterised by a Th-1 pattern of cytokines. In lepromatous disease there is a dominant Th-2 response with impaired cell-mediated immunity. Thus, patients with lepromatous disease have large numbers of bacilli in skin and nerve lesions and are anergic. Interferon-γ increases intracellular killing of mycobacteria. Although tuberculous meningitis is more common in HIV-infected individuals the attributable mortality is the same as seronegative patients. Corticosteroid use is a risk factor for the development of tuberculosis but are also used in some circumstances where the host response to infection is damaging, this includes tuberculous pericarditis and meningitis.

48. (a) T. Ventricular hypertrophy typically develops during the first two decades. It may involve both ventricles and the interventricular septum, with a reduction in internal chamber dimensions.
    (b) F. Familial HOCM variants are inherited in an autosomal dominant manner.
    (c) T. The primary genetic defects are in myocardial muscle proteins.

(d) T. The natural history of HOCM is variable, but it is an important cause of sudden death in young adults and the diagnosis may only be made at autopsy. Syncope may be arrhythmia-related, or due to a fall in stroke volume and blood pressure when the heart rate increases on exertion.

(e) T. Arterial pulses may, however, feel normal in character. A systolic murmur may be present internal to the apex. It is separated from the first sound, and starts later and louder than the symmetrical murmur of aortic stenosis.

49. (a) T.
    (b) T.
    (c) T.
    (d) F.
    (e) T.

Cystic fibrosis is a fatal autosomal recessive disorder most common in the caucasian population, with an incidence ranging from 1 in 2000 to 1 in 3000 live births. The classic form of the condition is clinically manifested by elevated concentrations of sweat electrolytes, pancreatic exocrine insufficiency, male infertility, obstructive pulmonary disease, and gastrointestinal tract obstruction. The molecular basis of the disease was discovered in 1989 with the identification of the defective CFTR gene on the long arm of chromosome 7. This spans approximately 230 kb, comprising 27 exons. The gene encodes a 170 kDa protein that functions as a cAMP regulated chloride channel on the apical surface of epithelial cells. The commonest mutation in cystic fibrosis is the delta 508 mutation, but other mutations of the CFTR gene may be found in patients with congenital absence of the vas deferens. However, around one fifth of patients with the latter condition do not carry any CFTR mutations.

There is increasing interest in the use of gene therapy in the disease, and both viral vectors and liposomes have been used as vectors to transfer the CFTR cDNA to the nucleus in affected patients, where it can compensate for the mutations in the two parental CFTR genes.

50. (a) T.
    (b) T.
    (c) T.
    (d) F.
    (e) T.

HIV-1-associated neurological disease affects 40–60% of patients with AIDS. Neuropathology attributed to the virus can be identified at autopsy in 9 out of 10 patients dying with AIDS.

In adults the commonest manifestation is HIV-1 dementia, which can result in motor defects, unsteady gait and tremor, behavioural changes, apathy and loss of libido and cognitive defects. In children HIV-1 encephalopathy occurs more commonly, and this is associated with impaired brain growth, motor deficits, and developmental impairment. Neuropathologically the condition may be manifest as an encephalitis, or a leukoencephalopathy. The former is associated with numerous foci of reactive microglia and disseminated multi-nucleated giant cells. Efficient productive HIV infection, resulting in the presence of detectable viral structural proteins in the cell, has been shown to occur only in cells of monocyte lineage (e.g. multi-nucleated giant cells, brain macrophages and microglia. It has not been demonstrated in cells of neuroectodermal origin such as astrocytes, neurones and oligodendrocytes. HIV-1 leukoencephalopathy is characterised by reactive astrocytosis, the presence of multi-nucleated giant cells, and white matter pallor. There is usually little or no inflammatory infiltrate.

A disorder of the spinal cord called 'vacuolar myelopathy' may also occur, and this is characterised by oedema surrounding myelinated fibres. There appears to be a preferential tropism of HIV-1 for sub-cortical regions of the CNS – the basal ganglia and pons, and cerebral white matter. MRI scanning in demented patients typically shows cerebral atrophy, ventricular enlargement, and numerous diffuse white matter abnormalities, but these features are not exclusive to HIV-1-related disease, and similar features, for example, may be found in patients with the primary anti-phospholipid syndrome. There are numerous potential neurotoxins in HIV-1 dementia, and there is experimental evidence that the HIV-1 GP120 molecule is itself neurotoxic, and may induce the production of soluble factors from microglia, and the expression of numerous cytokines have been shown to be elevated in patients with HIV-1 dementia, including TNF-α, IL-6 and PAF. Arachidonic acid metabolites are also present at elevated levels in HIV-1 dementia.

51. (a) F.
    (b) T.
    (c) F.

(d) T.
(e) T.
Mannose binding protein belongs to a group of proteins called the 'collectins'. The molecule is structurally similar to C1q, a bovine molecule called conglutinin, and the lung surfactant proteins A and D. All these proteins have a collagen-like region, hence the name collectin. The structure of C3 is quite dissimilar. Unlike C1q, mannose binding protein is synthesised by hepatocytes, and the gene encoding the protein is located on the long arm of chromosome 10. MBP is able to activate the classical complement pathway, independently of antibodies. Individuals with lower levels of the protein in the serum have defective opsonic capacity, and this results in an increased susceptibility to infection in infancy, particularly between 6 and 24 months of age. It has recently been shown that adults with partial deficiency are also more susceptible to infection. The MBP gene has regulatory features characteristic of acute phase proteins, and it has been shown that levels of the protein rise 3-fold in patients undergoing operations, or following acute malarial infection. The biological significance of these observations is not known.

52. (a) F.
    (b) F.
    (c) T.
    (d) T.
    (e) F.
Hepatitis C is a positive stranded RNA virus of 9379 nucleotides classified within the Flaviviridae. As yet there is no diagnostic test for hepatitis C viral antigens in human serum and therefore infection is usually diagnosed following detection of antibodies by immunoassay. The parenteral route is the most important route of transmission whilst transmission via saliva, human bite, sexual intercourse and mother to infant are all recorded in the literature. However, the route of infection is unclear in up to one third of cases. Infection may result in a spectrum of disease including acute hepatitis, chronic hepatitis, cirrhosis, vasculitis, and cryoglobulinaemia. In addition to supportive treatment, interferon-α and the guanosine analogue ribavirin, both alone and in combination, may have beneficial effects.

53. (a) F.
    (b) F.
    (c) T.
    (d) T.
    (e) T.
Polycythaemia is defined as an increase in the total red blood cell mass and using the isotope dilution method with erythrocytes labelled with ^{51}chromium values $>125\%$ are diagnostic. Polycythaemia should be monitored using the packed cell volume (PCV) rather than the haemoglobin concentration. This compensates for patients in which the haemoglobin is disproportionately low as a result of iron deficiency. If a patient requires venesection more than 3–4 times per year to maintain a stable PCV then cytotoxic therapy should be considered. Management by intensive venesection has been shown to significantly increase the risk of thrombotic complications. Hydroxyurea is now more commonly used than either busulphan and chlorambucil. Furthermore, hydroxyurea does not significantly increase the risk of leukaemic transformation in contrast to alkylating agents and radioactive phosphorous. There are numerous causes of polycythaemia including primary proliferative polycythaemia (polycythaemia rubra vera), secondary to hypoxia in chronic airflow limitation and cyanotic congenital heart disease, polycystic kidneys, renal neoplasms, cerebellar haemangioblastoma and uterine leiomyomata. Severe pseudo-polycythaemia may cccur in primary pulmonary hypertension.

54. (a) F.
    (b) T.
    (c) T.
    (d) T.
    (e) T.
Initially in HIV infection the lymph nodes are enlarged and histological examination reveals active germinal centres with HIV replication within the node. As the disease progresses the germinal centres become depleted of CD4 cells and the nodes become atrophic. Regression of lymphadenopathy is thus a bad sign in patients with HIV. Neopterin is a surrogate marker of HIV progression; it is a protein released by activated macrophages and predicts progression to AIDS independently of the CD4 count. Neopterin levels are also increased in opportunistic

infections associated with macrophage activation including tuberculosis. The MT-2 assay measures the ability of HIV strains to induce syncytia, that is fusion into giant cells, in T-cells. The syncytial-inducing strains are associated with more rapid disease progression. Active hepatitis B infection is associated with immune-activation and increased HIV replication and a decline in CD4 counts. Smoking is also associated with a poorer outcome although the mechanism is unclear.

55. (a) F.
     (b) T.
     (c) F.
     (d) F.
     (e) T.
     HLA B27 is a human class 1 MHC antigen which is found with greatly increased prevalence in patients with spondyloarthropathies, a group of disorders including reactive arthritis, spondylitis associated with inflammatory bowel disease or psoriasis, and ankylosing spondylitis. It is also associated with acute anterior uveitis. The arthritis which develops in affected patients following chlamydia infection or infection with Gram-negative organisms is a *reactive* one, and while bacterial antigens can in certain situations be isolated from the joint, whole organisms cannot be detected, and the arthritis which develops is not 'infective'. B27-positive patients are more frequently males, and show more peripheral disease, more 'bamboo spine' lesions, and more uveitis. In this patient group inflammatory bowel disease, psoriasis and erythema nodosum are generally less common than in B27 negative patients. Disease generally develops 10 years earlier in B27-positive patients. There have been extensive studies looking for associated disease susceptibility or severity genes on chromosome 6 and elsewhere, but no such associations have been found to date. It has no specific association with any TNF allele.

     HLA B27 is involved in the presentation of peptides to cytotoxic T lymphocytes, but these are generally composed of nine amino acids. Introduction of human HLA B27 with its associated light chain beta-2 microglobulin into rats, using transgenic techniques, results in the development of a spontaneous multi-system inflammatory disease bearing a strong clinical and histological resemblance to the human spondyloarthropathy. Local features include inflammatory bowel disease primarily affecting the colon, spondylitis, peripheral arthritis, and a variety of skin lesions and male genital inflammation. Trangenic mice are generally less severely affected, but are more susceptible to a naturally occurring ankylosing enthesopathy of the ankle and tarsal joints (ANKENT). The susceptibility to the disease in both rats and mice is related to the gene copy number.

56. (a) F.
     (b) T.
     (c) T.
     (d) F.
     (e) T.

Homocystinuria results from deficiency of cystathionine synthetase, resulting in the accumulation of homocystine, increased levels of urinary homocystine, and deficiency of cystine and cystathione. Clinical features of the syndrome include osteoporosis, recurrent arterial and venous thromboses, malar flush, and fair hair. Downward dislocation of the lens occurs, with myopia and cataracts. Many of the features of the syndrome resemble Marfan's, in that the patients are excessively tall, have long extremities, pectus excavatum, a scoliosis and a high-arched palate. Patients exhibit joint and ligamentous laxity, and may develop herniae. Hypermobility may pre-dispose to early degenerative arthritis, and vertebral osteoporosis may develop.

Patients may have a normal IQ, but in some affected individuals intelligence is reduced, resulting in learning difficulties. Unlike Marfan's syndrome, aortic root pathology and other valvular disease do not normally develop. The condition can be treated by dietary restriction of methionine, and oral pyridoxine and cysteine supplements may also be beneficial.

57. (a) F.
     (b) T.
     (c) F.
     (d) T.
     (e) F.

It is now clear that the endothelium plays a central role in the development of atherosclerotic plaques. Atheroma my be likened to a chronic inflammatory process in the tunica intima of large arteries probably initiated by endothelial damage. Low density lipoproteins (LDL) have been shown to activate endothelial cells and to induce the expression of adhesion molecules including

ICAM-1. The consequences of EC activation include the migration of monocytes from the bloodstream into the intima where they are transformed to foam cells following the uptake of LDL. Following a complicated sequence of events involving both t-PA and metalloproteinases the local smooth muscle cells are released from the media and proliferate locally. The atherosclerotic plaques that subsequently develop are located in the intimal layer.

58. (a) T.
    (b) F.
    (c) T.
    (d) T.
    (e) F.

The rheumatoid synovium in active disease represents a highly complex local environment of both cellular and soluble factors including a variety of cytokines. Cytokines have been measured in synovial fluid and synovial tissue in inflammatory and non-inflammatory diseases, and in normals. IL-1 and TNF co-exist in the rheumatoid joint and can induce the synthesis of each other by local macrophages and infiltrating monocytes. These cytokines stimulate the synthesis of metalloproteinases (collagenase, stromelysin and proteoglycanase) by chondrocytes, fibroblasts, macrophages and neutrophils resulting in local damage to bone, cartilage and proteoglycans. Interferon-γ is, somewhat surprisingly, not found in high concentration in synovial fluid in established disease. The control of inflammatory processes is not well understood. However there is evidence to suggest that transforming growth factor-β has an important regulatory role, and that both the IL-1 receptor antagonist and soluble TNF-receptors also contribute. The T cells that migrate into the rheumatoid synovium have been shown by flow-cytometric and histological analysis to be predominantly of the memory phenotype.

59. (a) F.
    (b) T.
    (c) F.
    (d) F.
    (e) T.

Primary syphilis arises at the site of inoculation after an incubation period of 21 days (3–90-day range). Painless regional lymphadenopathy is found in primary syphilis with generalised lymphadenopathy in secondary disease. Asymptomatic CNS invasion can be detected in some cases with primary infection and in at least 40–50% of those with secondary disease. Syphilis can be successfully treated in pregnancy with penicillin. Erythromycin may fail to treat syphilis in the fetus due to poor passage across the placenta. Treponema pallidum haemagluttination assay (TPHA) is specific for treponemal infection. False-positive reactions can occur with other spirochaetal infections such as yaws, lyme disease and leptospirosis. Venereal Disease Research Laboratory (VDRL) test is a non-treponemal (re-agenic) test based on the detection of IgG and IgM antibodies directed against cardiolipin. These are found as a result of infection with syphilis but biologic false-positive reactions may be found in other infections, autoimmune diseases and pregnancy.

60. (a) T. HLA is the most important genetic influence on the development of insulin-dependent diabetes. This has now been convincingly shown by a total genome screen for type I diabetes susceptibility genes.
(b) T. Examples of this combination are leprechaunism, Rabson–Mendenhall syndrome and the syndrome of type A insulin resistance.
(c) F. Although insulin receptor defects *can* cause NIDDM, these receptor defects account for less than 2% of cases of non-insulin dependent diabetes.
(d) True. While type II diabetes mellitus typically develops in middle-aged/older patients, 'maturity onset diabetes of the young' (MODY) is frequently due to genetic defects of glucokinase.
(e) T. Mitochondrial DNA is discussed further in Q. 34.

61. (a) F.
(b) T.
(c) F.
(d) F.
(e) F.
Anti-nuclear antibodies (ANA) are much loved by rheumatologists and are becoming increasingly useful in both diagnosis and estimation of prognosis in a variety of connective tissue disorders. The anti-nuclear antibody test is a screening test for autoimmune

disease and it must be borne in mind that many positive results are the result of drug therapy, old age, rheumatoid arthritis, chronic infection or association with organ-specific autoimmune diseases. Antibodies to extractable nuclear antigens (ENA) and generally more closely associated with disease than the ANA and may be positive when the ANA test is negative.

Antibodies to Sm are present in 5–30% of patients with systemic lupus erythematosus (SLE). The Jo-1 antigen is a tRNA histidyl synthetase and antibodies against Jo-1 are found in approximately 30% of patients with polymyositis. Antibodies to the ribonucleoprotein antigens Ro and La are found in 65% and 50%, respectively, of patients with primary Sjögren's syndrome and may also be found in patients with SLE. Anti-Ro antibodies in maternal serum may be associated with fetal congenital heart block. Anti-RNP antibodies are found in up to 25% of patients with SLE and less often in systemic sclerosis and polymyositis. Particularly high titres may be found in patients with mixed connective tissue disease, which is characterised by a combination of features including Raynaud's phenomenon, swollen fingers, and some of the features of SLE, scleroderma, myositis and rheumatoid arthritis.

62. (a) T.
    (b) T.
    (c) F.
    (d) T.
    (e) F.
    Following acute HIV infection there is generalised lymphopenia and a reduction in both CD4 and CD8 cells. The CD4 count may fall below 500 and opportunistic infections including PCP may occur in this period. In addition there is a high level of HIV replication and a high level of plasma viraemia making these patients more infectious than later in the course of disease. HIV viraemia is terminated by the onset of a cytotoxic CD8 T-cell response that is detectable before anti-HIV antibodies. Depending on the methods used, anti-HIV antibodies are detectable in the serum of over 90% of patients within 2 weeks of the onset of symptoms. Patients with a more prolonged and severe seroconversion illness have a worse prognosis.

63. (a) T. It is a neurotransmitter in both the peripheral and central nervous systems (where it is thought to be important for memory formation).

(b) T. Certain nitric oxide synthase enzymes may be activated by cytokines (see Q. 15 too).

(c) F. NO inhibits platelet aggregation.

(d) F. Nitric oxide is unstable and in solution forms toxic nitrite species. It can be delivered therapeutically into the lungs as a gas at low concentration mixed with oxygen. The avidity of haemoglobin for NO means that it is instantaneously delivered to vascular endothelium in the lung. This may be of benefit in both adult and neonatal respiratory distress syndromes and some forms of pulmonary hypertension.

(e) T. NO activates the enzyme guanylate cyclase.

64. (a) F.
    (b) T.
    (c) T.
    (d) T.
    (e) T.

Familial mediterranean fever is generally transmitted in an autosomal recessive manner. It can occur in many ethnic groups but is commonest in Jews, Turks and Armenians. It would be unusual for the condition to be manifest in childhood, and patients generally present as teenagers. Clinical features include polyarthritis, rash, myalgia, headaches, pericarditis, spleno-megaly, episcleritis, pleurisy. The commonest presenting feature is, however, abdominal pain.

The condition is characterised by a marked acute phase response, with high levels of IL-6, a high ESR, high CRP and the other features of cytokine-mediated activation of the immune system (e.g. hyperglobulinaemia, leukocytosis, raised fibrinogen). Attacks are generally self-limiting, lasting between 24 and 48 hours, and they may respond to the use of oral colchicine. This drug has also been used chronically to reduce the frequency of attacks.

Familial mediterranean fever may predispose to amyloid, and the use of agents to reduce attack frequency is under evaluation to see if it is possible to reduce the incidence of late amyloidosis. For reasons which are not understood, amyloid complicating FMF is commonest in patients of Sephardic Jewish origin.

65. (a) T.
    (b) F.
    (c) T.

(d) T.
(e) T.

Sulphasalazine is a chemical combination of sulphapyridine and 5-aminosalicylic acid (ASA). It is primarily used in the treatment of inflammatory bowel disease and rheumatoid arthritis. Activity resides primarily in the 5-ASA moiety, and sulphapyridine acts mainly as a carrier to the colonic site of action. Newer drugs are now available such as Mesalazine (5-ASA) and Olsalazine (two molecules of ASA bound together which separate in the large bowel), which do not have the sulphonamide-associated side-effects of sulphasalazine. The drug is of value in the treatment of ulcerative colitis particularly, but its value in small bowel disease in Crohn's is less well established. It is well tolerated in RA, and its use has been systematically evaluated in elderly patients, in whom it is well-tolerated.

The drug has a range of haematological side-effects including Heinz body anaemia, reversible neutropoenia, folate deficiency, thrombocytopoenia, agranulocytosis and aplastic anaemia. It may cause nausea, vomiting and epigastric pain, as well as headaches and dizziness and a rash. Pancreatitis, Stevens–Johnson syndrome, hepatitis, photosensitisation, and a lupus-like syndrome with a positive ANA have been described. Urine may be discoloured orange, and staining of contact lenses may also occur.

66. (a) T.
    (b) F.
    (c) T.
    (d) F.
    (e) T.

The relationships between genetic factors and autoimmune disease are well described. The only definite genetic factor so far described has been the HLA system. The associations between individual autoimmune diseases and different HLA antigens are too numerous to list but are well described in a variety of immunology and medical textbooks. Sjögren's syndrome is strongly associated with HLA DR3, and the linked genes B8 and DQ2, and the C4A null gene. Rheumatoid arthritis and pemphigus vulgaris are linked with HLA-DR4 whilst Good-pastures syndrome is associated with HLA DR2. Behçets syndrome is associated with a high prevalence of HLA B5 antigen in association with DR7 and DRw52.

67. (a) T.
    (b) T.
    (c) T.
    (d) T.
    (e) T.
    Whipple's disease is a rare condition described by George Whipple in 1907 and caused by the recently described organism *Tropheryma whippelii*. The disease is classically associated with staining of the organisms with the periodic acid Schiff reagent. However, the polymerase chain reaction now forms the basis of a sensitive diagnostic test. Ten percent of patients have neurological involvement at some stage during their disease. The most frequent neurological features include dementia, ophthalmoplegia and facial myoclonus and the nervous system is a common site of disease relapse. In the treatment of the condition it has been recommended that initial treatment should consist of parenteral penicillin and streptomycin for 2 weeks followed by co-trimoxazole for 1 year.

68. (a) T.
    (b) T.
    (c) F.
    (d) F.
    (e) F.
    A rare complication of varicella-zoster of the fifth cranial nerve is a necrotising cerebral vasculitis on the side of the lesion leading to a contralateral hemiparesis. Topical steroids are used in combination with anti-viral agents to reduce the corneal scarring produced by keratitis due to varicella-zoster. In contrast, topical steroids are contraindicated in corneal infections due to herpes simplex. The virus remains latent in the sensory (dorsal) nerve roots. Varicella pneumonia is very unusual in children unless they are immunosuppressed. Zoster-immune globulin (ZIG) is not effective beyond 72–96 hours after exposure. ZIG is a scarce resource and should be reserved for vulnerable hosts such as pregnant women and the immunosuppressed.

69. (a) T. A three base pair deletion in exon 10 of the CFTR (cystic fibrosis transmembrane conductance regulator) accounts for 70% of mutations in many Western and other populations. The deletion results in the loss of a phenylalanine at Codon 508 designated F508.

(b) T. See Q. 49 too.

(c) F. Antenatal screening uses the analysis of genomic DNA, so it is irrelevant whether the gene is expressed in foetal tissues.

(d) T. Cystic fibrosis is one of the commonest monogenic disorders in the population.

(e) T. As a general rule, successive generations are usually affected by dominant, rather than recessive disorders.

70. (a) T.
    (b) F.
    (c) F.
    (d) T.
    (e) T.

The term immunophilin refers to a series of proteins that serve as cellular receptors for three important immuno-suppressant drugs, cyclosporin A, FK506 and rapamycin. These molecules interact with a number of different signal transduction systems within the cell, and many of these are indeed calcium-dependent and dependent on phosphorylation pathways.

Levels of immunophilin in the brain are around 30 times higher than in other tissues. Cyclosporin A binds to the cylcophilin proteins, and FK506 binds to a specific binding protein FKBP. The immunophylins are all of low molecular weight, between 12 and 40 kDa. The effects of cyclosporin A–cyclophylin complexes and FK506–FKBP12 complexes are mediated via the calcium- and calmodulin-dependent protein phosphatase known as calcineurin. IL-2 gene transcription is predominantly regulated by a transcription factor of activated T cells called NFAT. The cytoplasmic component of this transcription factor must be translocated to the nucleus to influence the IL-2 gene. Phosphorylated NFAT is a calcineurin substrate, and treatment with FK506 can prevent translocation of NFAT to the nucleus, by inhibiting its dephosphorylation. FK506 can also enhance nitric oxide synthetase phosphorylation, and may have a role in inhibiting the toxicity of glutamate in the nervous system.

71. (a) F.
    (b) T.
    (c) F.
    (d) F.
    (e) T.

Heparin preparations initiate anti-coagulation rapidly, and have a short duration of action. Standard heparin is usually described as 'unfractionated', to distinguish it from low molecular weight heparins which generally have a longer duration of action. A number of low molecular weight preparations are available – Calciparin, Enoxaparin, and Tinzaparin, for example. They are given once daily sub-cutaneously, and may be self-administered in some circumstances.

These drugs are widely used in prophylaxis to reduce the risk of venous thrombosis following major orthopaedic surgery. The standard recommended prophylactic regimen for the commonly used Calciparin (Fragmin) preparation, is 2500 units 1–2 hours before surgery, followed by 2500 units every 24 hours for 5 days. The dose may be increased in high-risk patients. These preparations have a predictable dose–response relationship, and it is not usually necessary to monitor therapy with either the APTT or PT.

72. (a) T.
    (b) F.
    (c) T.
    (d) F.
    (e) F.
Sjögren's syndrome (SS) is a group of diseases characterised by inflammation and destruction of exocrine glands including lacrimal and salivary glands and occasionally pancreas, sweat glands, and mucus secreting glands of the bowel, vagina and bronchial tree. Sjögren's syndrome is strongly associated with HLA DR3, and the linked genes B8 and DQ2, and the C4A null gene. Antibodies to the ribonucleoprotein antigens Ro and La are found in 65% and 50% of patients with primary SS. Histological features of the damaged glands include dense epithelial MHC class II antigen expression and a mononuclear cell infiltrate consisting of 90% CD4+ T cells and 10% B cells. Renal complications are seen in 5–10% of SS patients with the commonest lesion being an interstitial nephritis +/- renal tubular acidosis type I (occasionally type II is seen). Occasionally patients develop an immune complex-mediated glomerulonephritis which is typically membranous. Finally, SS may complicate graft versus host disease.

73. (a) F.
    (b) T.
    (c) T.
    (d) F.
    (e) T.

The majority of immunodeficiency syndromes are inherited and usually present as recurrent or overwhelming infection in young children. However, some immunodeficiency syndromes are acquired and may present in adult life including the effects of drugs, irradiation or infection with HIV. Bruton's agammaglo-bulinaemia is the result of an X-linked deficiency. In patients with DiGeorge syndrome the thymic epithelium fails to develop normally and hence T cells cannot mature, and the result is that both T cell-dependent antibody production and cell-mediated immunity are much reduced. Wiskott–Aldrich syndrome is an X-linked defect resulting in an increased susceptibility to encapsulated bacteria. Bare lymphocyte syndrome is associated with failure of MHC class II expression and absent CD4+ T cells whilst adenosine deaminase deficiency results in a severe combined immunodeficiency phenotype.

74. (a) F.
    (b) T.
    (c) F.
    (d) T.
    (e) F.

HIV is a retrovirus but belongs to the Lentivirus family. This includes simian immunodeficiency virus (SIV), HIV-2, HTLV-1 and 2, feline immunodeficiency virus, visna and maedi viruses (infect sheep) and equine infectious anaemia virus. HIV-2 is endemic to West Africa and seems to have a lower propensity to cause immunodeficiency than HIV-1. Following infection with HIV DNA copies of the viral RNA are made by reverse transcriptase, these are transported to the cell nucleus and inserted into host DNA by HIV integrase. Protease inhibitors result in the production of non-infectious HIV particles but do not prevent incorporation into the genome. The V3 loop of the surface protein gp120 appears to be critical in cellular interactions and mutation of this loop alters the cellular tropism of the virus.

75. (a) T. RFLP stands for restriction fragment length polymorphism. An RFLP close to the diseased gene is usually co-inherited with the disease gene, and, particularly if two RFLPs on either side of the disease gene are available, may give high predictive value of the disease state.
(b) F. In diseases such as sickle cell disease and cystic fibrosis it may be reasonable to infer the mutation without DNA analysis of other family members.
(c) T. If, for example, an RFLP is several centiMorgans from the disease gene, genetic recombination between the RFLP and disease gene may cause a false-positive or a false-negative result.
(d) T. Chorionic villus sampling can be carried out earlier than amniocentesis and generally does not require lengthy cell culture which may be required with amniocentesis. This results in much earlier diagnosis with chorionic villus sampling.
(e) T. The expanded triplet repeat unit characteristic of Huntington's chorea can be detected directly from the analysis of chorionic villus samples.

76. (a) T.
(b) F.
(c) F.
(d) F.
(e) T.
SSPE may be diagnosed from the basis of clinical findings, and oligoclonal banding pattern in the CSF, periodic complexes on EEG, and histologically. Clinical features include behavioural and cognitive changes (stage 1 disease), myoclonic jerking, seizures, optic atrophy, and retinal disease. Dementia or dystonia may also occur, as well as cerebellar or long tract signs. Stage 2 and stage 3 disease is characterised by severe dementia, cortical blindness and the development of a persistent vegetative state. The mean age of onset is around eleven years, and the disease is three to four times commoner in boys. This is associated with serological evidence of previous measles infection, and antibodies are detectable in both serum and CSF. It may not always be possible, however, to elicit a reliable history of definite previous measles infection. Measles infection in early infancy (particularly aged less than one year) confers the greatest risk of developing SSPE. The absolute numbers of cases have fallen in populations where vaccination has been widely taken up, but the biological risk of an individual child developing SSPE after measles infection has risen,

reflecting a shift towards infection at a young age. There are no cases of SSPE developing after measles vaccination in a previously non-immune subject, and vaccination neither accelerates the development of SSPE, nor makes the disease worse.

77. (a) F.
    (b) F.
    (c) F.
    (d) T.
    (e) T.

Primary biliary cirrhosis is associated with the presence of anti-mitochondrial antibodies. Anti-Sm antibodies stands for anti-'Smith' (the first patient in whom they were described) and are commonly found in SLE. SLE is also associated with antibodies to double-stranded DNA, anti-Ro and anti-cardiolipin antibodies, as well as with antibodies to C1q, and rarely C1 esterase-inhibitor. Autoantibodies associated with polymyositis include anti-nuclear antibodies, and anti-aminoacyl-tRNA synthetase enzymes such as anti-Jo1. The systemic form of scleroderma is typically associated with anti-Scl 70 antibodies (anti-topoisomerase), and the CREST variant is associated with anti-centromere antibodies. Cold agglutinin disease is associated with anti-I antibodies.

78. (a) T.
    (b) T.
    (c) F.
    (d) T.
    (e) F.

Giardiasis is the most likely diagnosis in this man and is diagnosed by recognising the cysts in stools or the flagellate form in jejunal juice or mucus. Endoscopic intestinal biopsy and sampling is the most reliable way of establishing the diagnosis. Barium enema is not the investigation of choice in a patient with this history which suggests small bowel pathology. Folate deficiency is a common complication of small bowel malabsorption.

This history is not typical of typhoid fever where constipation is seen for the first 7–10 days and then replaced by diarrhoea. Metronidazole is the treatment of choice for *Giardia lamblia* infections and is given orally as 2 g per day for 3 days or 400 mg t.d.s. for 5 days. Alternative treatments include tinidazole and mepacrine hydrochloride.

79. (a) T.
    (b) F.
    (c) F.
    (d) F.
    (e) F.
    Tetracyclines bind the 30S subunit of bacterial ribosomes and block binding of tRNA to the A site of the ribosome. Rifampicin inhibits protein synthesis by an action on bacterial RNA polymerase. Quinolones act through inhibition of DNA gyrase. Glycopeptides (vancomycin and teicoplanin) act on the cell wall of Gram-positive bacteria inhibiting peptidoglycan synthesis. Imipenem is derived from the beta-lactam ring and like penicillins and cephalosporins inhibits transpeptidase enzymes (penicillin-binding proteins) involved in bacterial cell wall synthesis.

80. (a) F. The point here is that apoptosis ('programmed cell death') does not result in the release of intracellular substances which are toxic to surrounding cells. It has been described as an 'altruistic' process.
    (b) F. Cells typically shrink, rather than swell. A characteristic pattern of 'DNA-laddering' results if the intracellular contents are analysed on a gel.
    (c) T. Cells that do not find their target in the embryological development of the CNS die by apoptosis.
    (d) T. Programmed cell death of tumour cells in response to cytotoxic agents or irradiation is prevented or suppressed in cells with non-functional p53 genes.
    (e) F. When inhibitors of transcription are used in cell culture models, cells still undergo apoptosis. This indicates that the cell is synthesising the necessary molecules for programmed cell death constitutively.

81. (a) T.
    (b) T.
    (c) T.
    (d) T.
    (e) F.
    There are about 4 million diagnosed cases of Alzheimer's in the USA, and half a million in Britain. Certain genes for apo-lipoprotein E (Apo E) are associated with increased susceptibility to Alzheimer's. Both the risk of developing the condition, and

the age which the disease starts is influenced by whether a patient has 0, 1 or 2 copies of the epsilon 4 allele. However some elderly people with this gene have not developed the disease. The post-mortem appearance of the Alzheimer's brain is characterised by loss of neurones in certain cortical and sub-cortical areas, abundant neurofibrillary tangles and senile plaques which appear mainly in the grey matter. The tangles comprise paired helical filaments (PHFs) made from an unusual form of a protein which has a role in the stabilisation of cytoskeletal microtubules. There is increased deposition of insoluble β-AP, which is a peptide generated from β-amyloid precursor protein, encoded on chromosome 21. Down's patients have an extra copy of this chromosome, and have Alzheimer's disease in the majority of cases over the age of 30.

A number of drugs have been licensed for use in North America for the treatment of Alzheimer's including the hepatoxic drug tacrine. This is an inhibitor of acetylcholinesterase. Much research is going on into developing similar preparations, with improved therapeutic indices.

82. (a) T.
    (b) F.
    (c) F.
    (d) T.
    (e) F.
Acute inflammation has the characteristic phases: rubor, calor, tumor, dolor. Histologically acute inflammation is associated with infiltration by neutrophils, increased vascular permeability and local exudate formation. Therefore in an acute inflammatory lesion the up-regulation of endothelial cell adhesion molecules and the formation of a chemotactic gradient allows the influx of large numbers of neutrophils. In chronic inflammation there is on-going inflammation in the presence of healing and characteristically a mononuclear cell infiltrate consisting of lymphocytes, monocytes and giant cells.

Type IV hypersensitivity is a chronic inflammatory lesion, as seen for example, following intra-dermal PPD. Primary biliary cirrhosis is an example of chronic inflammation and granulomas may be seen in the liver biopsy.

83. (a) T.
    (b) F.

(c) T.
(d) F.
(e) F.
T lymphocytes express on their surface the CD3 antigen, which is closely associated with T-cell-receptor antigen. A subset of T lymphocytes are CD4 T-helper cells, the remaining lymphocytes are CD8-positive cytotoxic T cells. Memory T cells are characterised by the expression of the CD45 Ro antigen, whereas naive T cells express CD45 Ra as defined by monoclonal antibodies. Whilst T cells can produce IL-1, the predominant cytokine produced by T lymphocytes is interferon-γ. Lymphocytes are predominantly seen in type IV hypersensitivity reactions and not acute allergic reactions.

84. (a) T.
     (b) T.
     (c) F.
     (d) F.
     (e) T.
In legionella infections there is an initial neutrophil response (neutrophilia occurs in 70–80% of cases) but infection is controlled by cell-mediated immunity. Thus, patients with defects in cell-mediated immunity are at an increased risk of legionella. Smokers are also at increased risk and most fatalities occur in this group. *Mycoplasma pneumoniae* penetrates the respiratory epithelium alongside the cilia by binding to a surface glycoprotein but the organisms remain in the extracellular space. Mycoplasma infections are commonest in children and young adults and unlike other respiratory pathogens there is no increase in the elderly. *Coxiella burnetti* is transmitted by close contact with cattle and in addition to pneumonia, Q fever may present with hepatitis or endocarditis.

85. (a) T. G-proteins require the specific binding of an extracellular ligand to a cell membrane receptor.
     (b) T. There is evidence that structurally abnormal G-proteins are found in certain tumours, but the biological significance of these observations remains to be fully elucidated.
     (c) F. Steroid hormones are an important exception to the ubiquitous coupling of G-proteins and second messenger systems.

(d) F. Cholera toxin acts by inhibiting the inactivation of G_S (stimulatory G proteins) thus cAMP remains elevated and the intestinal epithelial cell secretes ions uncontrollably.

(e) F. The actions of G-proteins are most commonly confined to the cell membrane.

86. (a) T.
    (b) F.
    (c) F.
    (d) T.
    (e) F.

Particulate guanylate cyclase is a membrane-bound receptor with a binding site for both atrial and brain naturitic peptides. It has an internal catalytic domain which catalyses GTP to produce cyclic GMP.

Vascular smooth muscle has ATP-sensitive potassium channels, and the closure of these induced by ATP causes membrane depolarisation and calcium entry into cells. Drugs such as minoxidil and nicorandil which oppose the action of intracellular ATP on these potassium channels are vasodilators. Endothelin 1, on the other hand, belongs to the endothelin family of vasoactive peptides. Endothelin 1 is a very potent vasoconstrictor. It can also stimulate growth in renal mesangial cells, and vascular smooth muscle cells. Two main angiotensin-2 receptors subtypes have been identified – AT1 and AT2. It is the AT1 receptors which are thought to mediate the vascular actions of angiotensin 2, but the AT2 receptor sub-type is the most prevalent in human myocardial tissue. Angiotensin 2 inhibits renin release via the kidney, and this effect is mainly mediated through the AT1 receptor sub-type.

87. (a) T.
    (b) F.
    (c) T.
    (d) T.
    (e) F.

The circulation of T cells is now well described and naive T cells localise in secondary lymphoid organs until exposed to antigen. Memory T cells circulate through the tissues, such as the skin, screening for antigen and are smaller then naive T cells. All leukocytes express the adhesion molecule L-selectin, which is important in the initial tethering and rolling of leukocytes on endothelium, prior to transmigration into inflammatory lesions. The transmigration of leukocytes occurs across post-capillary venules and not small arterioles.

88. (a) F.
     (b) T.
     (c) T.
     (d) F.
     (e) T.
The toxins of cholera and diphtheria have a similar structure with A and B subunits. The B subunit interacts with the cell membrane allowing the active A subunit to enter the cell. The A subunit of the cholera toxin increases intracellular cyclic AMP leading to active secretion of chloride into the intestinal lumen.

   The diphtheria toxin inactivates elongation factor 2 which is essential for the interaction of tRNA with mRNA and, therefore, blocks protein synthesis. Botulinum neurotoxin acts pre-synaptically to prevent acetyl choline release. Pertussis toxin blocks signal transduction through an effect on G-proteins. Staphylococci associated with toxic shock syndrome produce a number of super-antigens including TSST-1.

89. (a) F.
     (b) F. The expression of Huntington messenger RNA is normal.
     (c) F. There is good evidence that in certain tissues the mutation continues to expand throughout life, which may help to explain some of the delayed onset effects.
     (d) T. The trinucleotide repeat expands between generations. If size correlates with severity/age of onset, which it seems to, this would explain why subsequent generations are affected earlier. This is what is meant by 'genetic anticipation'.
     (e) T. Fragile X syndrome is the most common form of heritable mental retardation (1:1500 male births) and is second only to Down's syndrome as a cause of moderate mental impairment in males. The name relates to a cytogenetic marker, a 'fragile site' on the X chromosome at Xq27.3 in which there is failure of the condensation of chromatin during mitosis.

90. (a) T.
     (b) F.

(c) T.
(d) F.
(e) F.

Hereditary haemorrhagic telangiectasia has recently been shown to be due to mutations in the gene encoding endoglin. This is a homodimerising transmembrane protein which binds TGF-β. This protein is produced by endothelial cells, and also occurs at high levels in placental tissues, particularly the syncytiotropho-blast. The precise pathological links between endoglin muta-tions, TGF-β function and the development of HHT remains to be elucidated. It is known that oestrogens increase TGF-β excretion from endothelial cells, and this phenomenon may be related to the tendency of pregnant women with the condition to develop life-threatening AV malformations during pregnancy which may bleed, or have adverse haemodynamic effects. In spite of the high level of endoglin in the placenta, the disease does not seem to be associated with an increased frequency of spontaneous abortion.

91. (a) F.
    (b) T.
    (c) F.
    (d) T.
    (e) F.

The endothelium is now known to have an active role and is involved in both acute and chronic inflammation, the main-tenance of vascular permeability, the clotting cascade, graft rejection, wound healing and the maintenance of vascular tone. During inflammation endothelial cells may produce and be activated by cytokines such as interleukin 1 and tumour necrosis factor (TNF), resulting in the expression of surface adhesion molecules and the production of tissue factor. Although activated by TNF endothelial cells themselves do not produce TNF which is largely produced by monocytes and macrophages. Endothelial cells are functionally heterogeneous with the most important features being found in the post-capillary venular endothelial cells. Although they play a role in chronic graft rejection, the endothelium is not involved in hyperacute graft rejection, which is principally the result of pre-formed antibodies.

92. (a) T.
    (b) F.

(c) F.
(d) F.
(e) T.
Parvovirus B19 also causes hydrops fetalis, acute arthritis in adults, aplastic crises in patients with haemolytic anaemia and chronic bone marrow infection in immunocompromised patients.

Chagas' disease is South American trypanosomiasis and is due to *T. cruzi*. Lyme disease is caused by *B. burgdorferi* and *B. recurrentis* is the cause of relapsing fever. *Chlamydia trachomatis* is the cause of lymphogranuloma venereum and chancroid is due to *H. ducreyi*.

Streptobacillus moniliformis is found in the mouths of rats and other rodents and produces a febrile illness with a petechial rash and in about half the cases an associated polyarthritis.

93. (a) F. The commonest inherited form of dwarfism is due to achondroplasia, an autosomal dominant disorder that often occurs as a new mutation.
(b) T. This condition is known as Laron dwarfism.
(c) T. The phenotype in achondroplasia is much more severe in homozygotes, who may not survive early infancy.
(d) T. The basis of achondroplasia has recently been determined at the molecular level, and in most cases a mutation in the receptor FGFR3 is implicated.
(e) F. Patients with achondroplasia are usually of normal intelligence.

94. (a) F.
(b) T.
(c) T.
(d) F.
(e) F.
Ondansetron is not a serotonin uptake inhibitor, but is a 5HT receptor type 3 antagonist. Ondansetron is used in the treatment of depression, and is a dopamine uptake inhibitor. Serotonin is a substrate for monoamine oxidase, and serotonin re-uptake inhibitors should not be used with MAO inhibitors.

The drug tacrine is an acetylcholinesterase inhibitor, and does cross the blood–brain barrier. It has been used in the USA for the treatment of patients with Alzheimer's disease.

Sumitriptan, used in the treatment of acute migraine, is a

powerful and selective 5-HT1-receptor agonist, but can cause chest pain due to coronary vaso-constriction, and is therefore contraindicated in patients with a previous history of ischaemic heart disease. Use with ergotamine should also be avoided.

95. (a) T.
    (b) F.
    (c) T.
    (d) T.
    (e) F.

Hypersensitivity is the term used to describe immune-mediated tissue damage. Many hypersensitivity reactions are mixed responses, but the original classification suggested by Coombs and Gell over 20 years ago, still provides a useful framework.

Type 1 reactions are elicited by the interaction of antigen with tissue mast cells or basophils passively sensitised with reagenic antibodies. In man, reactions of this type are IgE-mediated, and the local consequences of type 1 reactions are mediated by histamine, SRSA, and a range of other phlogistic mediators.

Type 2 reactions are initiated by antibody reacting with antigen which is part of the cell membrane, or with antigens that become cell associated. Examples of type 2 reactions are acute haemolysis as a consequence of incompatible blood transfusion, certain auto-immune haemolytic anaemias, and many drug-induced anaemias, such as those caused by α-methyldopa. The antibodies mediating type 2 reactions are typically complement fixing.

Immune complex-mediated hypersensitivity is classified as type 3. This may be manifest as serum sickness in patients exposed to antigens to which they have been previously sensitised. This type of reaction may occur with exogenous drug administration, e.g. with streptokinase, or anti-lymphocyte globulin, or may occur following exposure to a virus. Dengue haemorrhagic shock in man is an example of the latter. Severe haemorrhagic complications of Dengue infection occur more frequently in pre-sensitised individuals, as a consequence of a type 3 hypersensitivity reaction. Type 4 hypersensitivity reactions are mediated by antigen specific T cells, which release lymphokines attracting other inflammatory cells, particularly macrophages. Antibody and complement are not necessary, though many examples of hypersensitivity reactions seen clinically are mixed, and antibodies may also be involved.

96. (a) T.
    (b) F.
    (c) F.
    (d) T.
    (e) F.
    There are two types of twins, monozygotic and dizygotic. Comparison of concordance rates in monozygotic and dizygotic twins is a standard method used for comparison of the effects of genes and environment. If monozygotic pairs are not totally concordant for given trait, genetic factors alone cannot account for that trait. Monozygotic twins derive from a single zygote that divides very early in embryogenesis, generally within a week of fertilisation.

    While the incidence of monozygotic twinning is uniform in all populations, about 1:250–300 births, there is considerable racial variation in the incidence of dizygotic twinning. Dizygotic twins occur in about 1:500 Asians, and at a frequency of 1:20 in some African populations. Frequency in caucasians is around 1:125. It has been suggested there is a relationship with the maternal level of FSH, and multiple births are more common in patients treated with clomiphene citrate. A tendency to dizygotic twinning is familial, and the recurrent risk in families is quoted to be two to four times that in the general population.

    Two-thirds of monozygotic twins share a single chorion and common circulation, while dizygotic twins will invariably have two chorions. In dizygotic twins a single placenta is found in 40% of cases, and two placentae in 60%.

97. (a) T.
    (b) T.
    (c) T.
    (d) F.
    (e) T.
    Endothelial cell activation leads to morphological change and an increase in vascular permeability, which allows the formation of an exudate in acute inflammation. Activation of the endothelium with interferon-γ results in the expression on the surface of class II MHC antigens, which may play a role in antigen presentation. Endothelial cell activation also results in the release of nitric oxide, which results in local vascular dilatation and increased blood flow to areas of inflammation. Cytokine activation promotes a pro-coagulant state on the endothelial cell surface by increasing tissue factor activity and plasminogen activator

inhibitor, and by also decreasing prostaglandin I_2 release and thrombomodulin activity. Endothelial cell activation also results in cytokine release, principally interleukin-1β.

98. (a) T.
    (b) T.
    (c) T.
    (d) F.
    (e) T.
Cytokines are pleiomorphic, low molecular weight glycoproteins, which may be produced by a range of cells. Monocytes and macrophages are particularly good cytokine producers and produce interleukin 1 and 6 and TNF. Interferon-γ is predominantly produced by activated T lymphocytes and may increase the expression of MHC class II on monocytes.

Interleukin 2 has been used as an adjuvant prior to chemotherapy in various tumours and one of the side-effects of this is a systemic vascular leak syndrome, principally due to a direct toxic effect on endothelial cells. There is increasing interest in the use of both cytokines and their various antagonists in the treatment of a variety of diseases and a number of clinical trials are in progress.

99. (a) T.
    (b) T.
    (c) F.
    (d) T.
    (e) T.
After injection by a female anopheline mosquito, sporozoites from all forms of malaria invade the liver. After replication these form hepatic shizonts which rupture releasing merozoites into the circulation to infect erythrocytes. In *P. falciparum* and *P. malariae* the hepatic forms mature at the same time and there are no persistent liver parasites. In *P. vivax* and *P. ovale* some of the hepatic forms may persist and treatment with primaquine is required to eradicate the latent hepatic shizonts.

People lacking the Duffy red cell antigen are resistant to infection with *P. vivax*. *Plasmodium vivax* and *P. ovale* can only infect young erythrocytes and *P. malariae* can only infect old cells. *P. falciparum*, however, can infect erythrocytes of all ages which contributes to the severity of *P. falciparum* infection. Nephrotic syndrome is seen in *P. malariae* but in none of the other species.

The trophozoite form of the malaria parasite is responsible for asexual replication and rupture of erythrocytes leading to the manifestations of disease and is killed by anti-malaria treatment. The gametocytes are not cleared by quinine but must undergo sexual reproduction in a mosquito to produce infection and, therefore, persistent gametocytes do not indicate therapeutic failure.

100. (a) F. Obesity is rarely inherited as a simple Mendelian trait.
(b)/(c) F./T. Leptin is the gene product of the *obese* gene recently cloned from the *obese* mouse, and found to be conserved in humans. Leptin is secreted into the blood from adipose tissue and acts centrally as a satiety factor. Humans with obesity have been generally found to have raised blood leptin concentrations. Deficient leptin production is therefore thought to be an infrequent cause of human obesity; resistance to leptin action may be more common but is as yet unproven.
(d) T.
(e) F. MODY is an autosomal dominant condition and in at least 60% of cases is caused by glucokinase gene mutations. Obesity is generally not the major feature of MODY but is important in the cause of type 2 (non-insulin-dependent) diabetes occurring in older age groups.

101. (a) T.
(b) F.
(c) T.
(d) F.
(e) F.
Ibuprofen is generally thought to have fewer gastrointestinal side-effects than other non-steroidals, but this may be partly related to the fact that it is generally used in lower doses than many similar medications.
Azapropazone is associated with a high risk of gastrointestinal side-effects, and should not be used in elderly patients, or patients with a previous history of peptic ulceration. Piroxicam, ketoprofen, indomethacin, naproxen and diclofenac are associated with intermediate risks. Diclofenac may cause perturbation of liver function tests, and care is needed in the chronic administration of this drug, particularly in patients who are also receiving other hepatoxic agents such as methotrexate.
Tenoxicam has a long plasma half life (72 hours) and it takes 7–10 days to reach steady therapeutic blood levels using the

standard 20 mg dose. It makes it less attractive than other quicker acting non-steroidals in the management of acute gout. The use of such a drug is not appropriate in the long-term management of patients with severe osteoarthritis of the hips, in whom the treatment of choice is usually surgical. Phenylbutazone does have a role in the treatment of ankylosing spondylitis in a few patients, but is now restricted to patients under the care of hospital-based physicians. In addition to its gastric side-effects, it can cause severe fluid retention and may precipitate heart failure, and may also cause life-threatening agranulocytosis or aplastic anaemia, which can occur very acutely. It cannot therefore be described as a 'drug of choice' for the management of ankylosing spondylitis.

102. (a) T.
     (b) T.
     (c) F.
     (d) T.
     (e) F.

Factor V_{Leiden} results in activated protein C resistance. The mutation is a substitution of Arg 506 by Gln in the factor V gene, and has been recognised as a major cause of thrombophilia. The mutation is found in 2–7% of the normal population, and in 20–60% of patients who develop deep venous thrombosis. The mutation is associated with increased risk of thrombosis in patients taking the oral contraceptive pill, but does not confer increased risk in patients who have antiphospholipid antibodies. Affected patients can be detected by functional measurements for activated protein C resistance, or by genotypic analysis, usually using PCR-based methods. The latter rely on analysis of the patient's DNA, and are unaffected by the use of warfarin, or similar drugs.

103. (a) T.
     (b) T.
     (c) F.
     (d) T.
     (e) T.

Both interleukin 1 and interleukin 6 are implicated in the induction of the acute-phase response in diseases such as giant cell arteritis, polymyalgia rheumatica and multiple myeloma. A raised interleukin 6 level results in a high C reactive protein, a normocytic normochromic anaemia and a raised platelet count. Anti-cytokine antibodies are now being used in drug-trials of various diseases and antibodies against TNF have been shown to be effective in rheumatoid arthritis. Treatment with soluble TNF receptors in septic shock shows benefit in Phase II trials. The interferons have been used in a variety of diseases, including recurrent laryngeal papillomas, renal cell carcinoma and in the treatment of hepatitis C infection. Their treatment is limited by the side-effects, principally malaise and flu-like symptoms.

104. (a) T.
     (b) T.
     (c) F.
     (d) F.
     (e) F.
Primary infection with *Histoplasma capsulatum* presents with erythema nodosum (EN) and miliary shadowing on chest X-ray. Other manifestations of histoplamosis include calcified mediastinal lymph nodes, mediastinal fibrosis and disseminated disease in the immunocompromised host. A proportion of patients with leprosy experience a severe hypersensitivity reaction including EN, known as erythema nodosum leprae. Pontiac fever is a systemic illness due to *Legionella pneumophilia* and EN is not a feature. Primary tuberculosis is associated with EN which is rarely, if ever, encountered in reactivation disease. EN may follow streptococcal infections but there is no association with staphylococci.

105. (a) F. Like most enzyme defects, Gaucher's disease, a lysosomal storage disorder, is inherited as a recessive trait.
     (b) T. The substrate for the enzyme is a complex lipid normally degraded in the lysosome.
     (c) F. In Gaucher's disease there is an accumulation of glucocerebroside in the reticuloendothelial system, notably in the liver and spleen. Bone marrow replacement by lipid-laden macrophages ('Gaucher cells') occurs, compromising haematopoiesis. Bone marrow transplantation has been used to treat the disease and clinical trials of gene therapy have recently begun.
     (d) T. This is also true for several other recessive enzyme defects such as Tay-Sachs disease.
     (e) T.

106. (a) T.
  (b) F.
  (c) F.
  (d) F.
  (e) T.

Hepatitis B vaccination is recommended in doctors, dentists, nurses, midwives and others who are likely to come directly in contact with patients or their body fluids. Laboratory staff who come into contact with blood or blood products should also be vaccinated.

The most commonly used vaccine is now one containing hepatitis B surface antigen produced using a recombinant DNA technique. The vaccine is generally stored between 2° and 8° C and should be administered in normal subjects by the intramuscular route. Intradermal, or sub-cutaneous administration may be considered in patients with haemophilia. It is usually recommended that recipients of the vaccine be tested for the production of antibody between 2 and 6 months after administration. Full immunity can take up to 6 months to develop, and up to 15% of patients over the age of 40 do not respond.

Patients on long-term haemodialysis sero-convert poorly, and it is inappropriate to administer the vaccine in patients with deteriorating renal function, before they develop end-stage disease. The vaccine should not be administered to patients who are known to be hepatitis B surface antigen positive, or to patients with acute infection with the virus. The most common adverse reaction in normal subjects is local discomfort and erythema, but arthralgia and myalgia, have occasionally been described.

107. (a) F.
  (b) T.
  (c) T.
  (d) T.
  (e) T.

Knowledge of cellular adhesion molecules is becoming increasingly important in the study of inflammatory disease, malignant disease and graft rejection. The β2-integrins are made up of an α and a β chain and include lymphocyte function associated antigen-1 (LFA-1) and Mac 1. They are important in the adhesion of leukocytes to endothelium, and bind to intercellular adhesion molecule-1 (ICAM-1), ICAM-2 and ICAM-3. The selectins, E selectin and P-selectin expressed on endothelial cells and L selectin on leukocytes, mediate the initial tethering and subsequent rolling of leukocytes on endothelium in the initial stages of inflammation. ICAM-1 is intimately involved as a co-stimulatory molecule in the immune response and in the binding of T-cells to antigen-presenting cells. The circulating form of adhesion molecules have been measured in the serum in a variety of diseases and ICAM-1 has been shown to be raised in rheumatoid arthritis. In addition, ICAM-1 has been shown to be the receptor for both the *Plasmodium falciparum* malarial parasite and for rhinoviruses.

108. (a) T.
      (b) F.
      (c) T.
      (d) T.
      (e) T.
The immunoglobulin superfamily consists of a large number of molecules mainly involved in intercellular adhesion. All the members of the superfamily are related in structure to immunoglobulins and have a variable number of immuno-globulin domains. The selectins, P selectin, E selectin and L selectin form a separate group of single-chain glycoproteins and function as described above. ICAM-1 and VCAM-1 are both members of the immunoglobulin superfamily and are involved in leukocyte adhesion to endothelial cells, whilst CD2 is the ligand for LFA 3 and is important in lymphocyte interaction. Other members of the family include CD4, CD8, and MHC class I and class II.

109. (a) F.
      (b) T.
      (c) T.
      (d) F.
      (e) T.
ACE inhibitors inhibit the feedback mechanisms suppressing plasma renin levels. Plasma renin levels are therefore increased in patients receiving these drugs. Beta-blockers inhibit the secretion of renin stimulated by the sympathetic nervous system. ACE inhibitors reduce mortality of both after myocardial infarction and in patients with congestive cardiac failure.

There is reduced renal blood flow in renal artery stenosis, stimulating renin secretion. This in turn leads to high levels of angiotensin 2 which drives the hypertension. The use of an ACE inhibitor to inhibit angiotensin 2 will reduce blood pressure. Losartan is a specific angiotensin 2 receptor antagonist with properties similar to those of ACE inhibitors. However, it does not inhibit the breakdown of bradykinin and other vasoactive kinins, and does not cause the persistent cough which complicates therapy with ACE inhibitors.

A symptom complex has been described for ACE inhibitors which may include serositis, vasculitis, muscle pain, arthralgia, fever and a positive anti-nuclear antibody and raised ESR. Some patients develop a leukocytosis, and rashes, and photosensitivity reactions are not uncommon with these drugs.

110. (a) T.
　　(b) F.
　　(c) T.
　　(d) T.
　　(e) T.

By the sixth week of embryologic development in both sexes, the primordial germ cells have migrated to the gonadal ridges, where they are surrounded by the sex cords, forming a pair of primitive gonads. Whether chromosomally XX or XY, the developing gonad up until this time is bipotential. In the presence of a Y chromosome, the medullary tissue forms typical testes with Leydig cells and seminiferous tubules. Under the stimulation of HCG from the placenta, the male gonad develops the capacity to secrete androgens. The spermatagonia derive from the seminiferous tubules together with supporting Sertoli cells. The production of androgens by the Leydig cells of the fetal testes stimulates the mesonephric ducts to form the male genital ducts. The Sertoli cells produce a hormone that suppresses the formation of the paramesonephric (Mullerian) ducts.

During meiosis in the male, the X and Y chromosomes normally pair by segments at the ends of their short arms, in which region they undergo recombination. The sequences in the pseudo-autosomal region of the X and Y chromosomes normally exchange in meiosis 1. However, in rare cases genetic recombination can occur between the X and Y short arms outside the pseudo-autosomal region, and this abnormal exchange mechanism can produce XX males and XY females.

XX males have a 46 XX karyotype and usually possess some Y chromosomal sequences translocated to the short arm of the X chromosome. In phenotypic females with a 46 XY karyotype, there is loss of the testes-determining region of the Y chromosome. These sex reversal disorders occur in a frequency of around 1:20 000 births, but by far the most common sex chromosome defects in live-born infants and fetuses are the trisomic types – XXY, XXX and XYY. All three of these are rare in spontaneous abortions. Monosomy for the X chromosome (Turner syndrome), is relatively rare in live-born infants (phenotype frequency = 1:5000 live female births), but is the most common chromosome abnormality reported in spontaneous abortions.

In normal females, there is inactivation of one X chromosome. This does not occur in males, and the expression of X-linked genes is equalized between the two sexes. X inactivation is normally random in female somatic cells, though in patients with structural abnormalities of an X chromosome, the structurally abnormal chromosome is preferentially inactivated. Non-random inactivation is also observed in the case of X: autosome translocation. Patients with Kleinfelter's syndrome have the karyotype 47, XXY in most cases, though about 15% of patients have mosaic karyotypes. Others have been reported including 48 XXYY, 48 XXXY, and 49 XXXXY. Typically patients are tall thin males, and may appear physically normal until puberty. This occurs at the normal age, but testicular size is reduced. Gynaecomastia may or may not occur. Most patients have educational problems, and frequently poor psycho-social adjustment.

111. (a) T.
    (b) T.
    (c) F.
    (d) T.
    (e) F.

Leukocyte adhesion deficiency is an inherited immunodeficiency disease. The abnormality is the consequence of mutations in the CD18-β sub-set of the β2 integrins which prevents surface expression of all three CD18 integrins on leukocytes. The disease has been described in humans, dogs and cattle, and results in severe, life-threatening bacterial infections. The circulating neutrophil count is markedly raised due to a reduced marginating pool and an increased neutrophil life-span. The lack of the β2 integrins prevents neutrophil transmigration from the blood stream, across the endothelium into inflammatory sites in the tissues. Two separate types of leukocyte adhesion deficiency are now described: type 1 is an integrin deficiency and type 2 a selectin ligand deficiency.

112. (a) T.
    (b) F.
    (c) F.
    (d) F.
    (e) F.

Monoclonal antibodies originally described by Köhler and Milstein are now widely used in laboratories and are finding their way into clinical practice. The hybridomas used to produce monoclonals arise from a single cell and the resulting antibody therefore binds specifically to a single antigen. The hybridomas are produced by the fusion of antibody-producing plasma cells and an immortal myeloma line. The resultant hybridomas are then serially diluted and single cells cultured to produce the hybridoma lines. Monoclonal antibodies may be one of the IgG sub-classes or IgM and have a divalent structure unless experimentally modified. Monoclonal antibodies may be of mouse, rat or human origin.

113. (a) F.
    (b) T.
    (c) T.
    (d) F.
    (e) T.

HTLV-1 is associated with adult T-cell lymphoma, polymyositis and tropical spastic paraparesis. Ninety percent of cases of lymphoma in immunocompromised patients contain EBV-transformed cells. There is no proven association between EBV and chronic fatigue. Hantaan viruses are responsible for outbreaks of 'rodent-borne nephropathy'. These include haemorrhagic fever with renal syndrome in S. E. Asia and nephropathia epidemica in Northern Europe. More recently new strains of Hantaan have been described in the USA that produce an illness similar to the adult respiratory distress syndrome. Anal carcinoma, cervical carcinoma and carcinoma of the penis are all associated with human papilloma viruses.

114. (a) T.
    (b) T.
    (c) T.
    (d) F.
    (e) T.
    Brucella abortus (cattle) and *B. meletensis* (goats) are transmitted by milk and dairy products. Bartonellosis (Oroya fever) is due to infection with a Gram-negative rod: *Bartonella bacilliformis*. It is transmitted by New World sandflies and is limited to Central and South America. Dengue fever is spread by the *Aedes aegypti* mosquito. Aspergillus spores are inhaled and are present in marijuana. Outbreaks of aspergillosis in immunocompromised patients have been described in association with marijuana use and also building construction.

115. (a) F. It is an autosomal dominant genetic disorder (see also Q. 90).
    (b) T. These may occur either because of emboli from the lung, or because of primary lesions in the brain.
    (c) F. Recurrent GI haemorrhages occur in many patients.
    (d) T. This is frequently the treatment of choice, and highly selective angiography, combined with new sophisticated embolisation techniques, have revolutionised the therapy of HHT.
    (e) F. The penetrance is high, though variable, and the disease is clinically apparent in most children in the first decade.

116. (a) T.
    (b) F.
    (c) T.
    (d) T.
    (e) F.
    Monoclonal antibodies are being increasingly used in clinical practice. For example in haematology practice they have been used to deplete patient bone-marrow samples of malignant cells, and in stem-cell bone-marrow transplants to purify the pluripotential stem cells from the bone-marrow. In rheumatoid arthritis systemic treatment with monoclonal antibodies against TNF, ICAM-1 and CD4 have been used successfully in clinical trials. The main problem with the use of murine monoclonal antibodies in clinical practice has been the development of anti-mouse antibodies and this has been improved, to some extent, by humanising the antibody by the replacement of the murine

constant region with a human equivalent. Considerable research interest is focused on creating non-immunogenic antibody preparations for use in clinical practice.

117. (a) T.
     (b) F.
     (c) F.
     (d) F.
     (e) T.
Ancylostoma is also known as hookworm and is a major cause of iron-deficiency. IL-5 is the cytokine largely responsible for eosinophil recruitment. IL-6 is one of the mediators of the acute-phase response. Oncocerciasis (river blindness) is a form of filariasis but the microfilariae are found in the skin and are absent from the blood. Oncocerciasis is diagnosed by examining skin snip preparations. *Loa loa, Wucheria bancrofti* and *Brugia malayi* are the other main filaria and are found in blood films. *Taenia sagginatum* is the beef tapeworm, *T. solium* is the pork tapeworm responsible for cystercicosis.

   Trichinella spiralis is the cause of trichinosis, characterised by fever, myalgia and diarrhoea. The larvae migrate to skeletal muscle and the disease is transmitted by ingestion of poorly-cooked meat.

118. (a) T. Scrapie is a disease of sheep, and BSE, at the time of writing, at least, is not definitely known to be transmissable to humans (see also Q. 39). However, there have been a number of patients described recently in whom a CJD variant has been described, developing in younger subjects. This has been linked with BSE.
     (b) F. Prion particles, unlike viruses, are exclusively composed of protein.
     (c) F. It is rare in these age groups. CJD occurs in both sexes, mainly between the ages of 50 and 65 years.
     (d) T. The histological picture in the brain in CJD involves extensive neuronal degeneration, astrocytic proliferation and the characteristic development of minute vesicles in both neurones and glial cells – the so-called 'spongy' change, similar to that in BSE.
     (e) F. Kuru is due to cannibalism and its worldwide incidence is decreasing. It was originally described in the Fore people of New Guinea.

119. (a) T.
  (b) F.
  (c) F.
  (d) T.
  (e) T.
Deficiency of glucose-6-phosphate dehydrogenase is the commonest disease-producing enzyme defect in man. Over 300 variants are described, and one allele, the A variant occurs in 1:20 black males in America. G6PD deficiency confers some protection against malaria, and this is the commonly adduced explanation for the high gene frequency of G6PD variants in some populations. The normal variant of the enzyme is called the B type, which has normal electrophoretic mobility. The B⁻ variant has normal electrophoretic mobility but only 4% of normal enzyme activity, and occurs commonly in the Mediterranean regions. The A variant occurs in 20% of American black males, and is associated with around 90% of normal enzyme activity, and the A⁻ variant, occurring in 10% of American black males, results in only 15% enzyme activity. Around 1:500 American black females are genetically A⁻/A⁻, and are susceptible to drug-induced haemolytic anaemia. The A⁻ variant has decreased stability, but it is the reduced enzymic activity of the abnormal G6PD variants, which results in decreased production of NADPH, the major source of reducing equivalents in the erythrocytes. NADPH protects the cell against oxidative damage by the regeneration of reduced glutathione from the oxidised form. The defect originally came to attention with the use of the anti-malarial drug primaquine. Haemolysis can also occur following the use of sulphonamide antibiotics or dapsone, and following exposure to naphthaline. Enzyme defects also result in susceptibility to the oxidants in fava beans (*Vicia fava*).

120. (a) F.
  (b) T.
  (c) T.
  (d) F.
  (e) T.
The acetylation polymorphism was first discovered during treatment of patients with tuberculosis with isoniazid. Slow acetylators are homozygous for a recessive gene, and rapid inactivators are homozygous for the normal variant or

heterozygous. The relevant enzyme is hepatic arylamine N-acetyltransferase, which is the product of a gene mapping to chromosome 8. Rapid acetylators have reduced enzyme levels. The frequency of the two alleles varies considerably in different ethnic groups. The slow acetylation phenotype is found in a minority of Asians (5–20%), while up to 65% of caucasians and 50% of American blacks are slow acetylator homozygotes. The rapid acetylator phenotype is most common in Eskimos and Japanese (95%). Toxicity with isoniazid therapy for tuberculosis occurs most commonly in slow acetylators, while historically, treatment failure sometimes occurred in rapid acetylators, particularly when the drug was given only once or twice weekly.

Other drugs which are metabolised by this pathway include procainamide, hydralazine, phenelzine and sulphonamides. It has been suggested that patients are more likely to develop procainamide or hydralazine induced lupus if they are slow acetylators. Acetylator status can be determined from a single urine sample following consumption of a beverage containing caffeine.

121. (a) F.
 (b) F.
 (c) T.
 (d) T.
 (e) F.
Serum cholinesterase (formerly called pseudo-cholinesterase) is an enzyme in human plasma that hydrolyses choline esters such as acetylcholine. The commonly used muscle relaxant succinylcholine (suxamethonium) comprises two molecules of succinylcholine and is normally hydrolized by cholinesterase, reducing the availability of succinylcholine at the motor end plate. Around 1:3000 individuals in European populations is homozygous for an atypical cholinesterase allele.

Affected individuals are unable to degrade succinylcholine at the normal rate, and prolonged apnoea requiring artificial ventilation may persist from one to several hours. Serum cholinesterase phenotypes cannot be determined reliably on the basis of enzyme levels in the serum, because there is great variation in the normal population. Sensitivity of testing can be increased by using alternative choline substrates, and a cholinesterase inhibitor such as dibucaine.

The allele frequency of the atypical allele which results in the succinylcholine sensitive homozygous phenotype is 0.017 in the population. The genetic defect is an Asp to Gly substitution at position 70. Other variants have been described such as the K variant, which occurs with an allele frequency of 0.113, and is due to an Ala to Thr substitution at position 539. Individuals homozygous for this variant have normal succinylcholine metabolism. Malignant hyperthermia is an autosomal dominant disorder, which results in an adverse response to muscle relaxants and inhalational anaesthetics. This is related to a genetically determined defect in intramuscular calcium handling, and is not due to an abnormality in serum cholinesterase.

122. (a) F.
     (b) T.
     (c) T.
     (d) F.
     (e) T.
Apoptosis, or programmed cell death, is now increasingly well-described. The differentiated cells of multi-cellular organisms all appear to share the ability to carry out their own death through activation of an internally encoded suicide programme. When activated this programme initiates a characteristic form of cell death called apoptosis. This can be triggered by a variety of extrinsic and intrinsic signals. Apoptotic cell death can be distinguished from necrotic cell death. Necrotic cell death is a pathologic form, resulting from acute cellular injury, typified by rapid cell swelling and lysis. Apoptosis is characterised by controlled auto-digestion of the cells, with cyto-skeletal disruption and cell shrinkage. The nucleus undergoes condensation and degradation.
   Autoimmune disorders, such as SLE and immune-mediated glomerulo-nephritis are associated with the inhibition of apoptosis, as are some cancers such as follicular lymphomas, breast and prostate cancer. Some chemotherapeutic drugs, such as cisplatin, doxarubicin, methotrexate and vincristine have been shown to induce apoptosis.

123. (a) F.
     (b) T.
     (c) T.
     (d) T.
     (e) T.

The key vascular change in sepsis is profound peripheral vasodilatation with a fall in systemic vascular resistance. Cardiac index is the cardiac output corrected for body surface area and is increased in most patients with sepsis. However, the rise in cardiac index is usually insufficient to compensate for the fall in systemic vascular resistance and hypotension results. In addition to poor oxygen delivery there is a failure of oxygen extraction from the circulation in sepsis due to shunting through capillary beds and local tissue hypoxia. This hypoxia leads to the lactic acidosis that accompanies severe sepsis and further impairs tissue function.

Echthyma gangrenosum is a characteristic necrotic skin lesion that is found in neutropenic patients with sepsis due to *Pseudomonas aeruginosa*.

124. (a) T. The lupus anticoagulant and antiphospholipid antibodies, particularly anticardiolipin antibodies are associated with arterial or venous thromboses, thrombocytopoenia and recurrent fetal loss.
(b) T. This gene defect is known as factor V_{Leiden} (see Q. 102).
(c) T. It should be remembered that Warfarin therapy profoundly affects many clotting parameters, and interpretation of a 'thrombophilia screen' on therapy may be difficult. Functional resistance to protein C is due to the factor V_{Leiden} mutation.
(d) T. A significant proportion of such cases will have an identifiable coagulation defect and may require long-term treatment. Study of other family members may be indicated.
(e) T. Patients with venous thromboembolism and arterial embolism have increased homocysteine levels after methionine loading. Patients with severe hyperhomocysteinaemia due to cystathionine-β synthase deficiency and methylene tetrahydrofolate reductase deficiency are also predisposed to venous and arterial thromboses.

125. (a) F.
(b) F.
(c) T.
(d) T.
(e) F.
The major histocompatibility complex in man is a complex locus composed of a large cluster of genes which are located on

the short arm of chromosome 6. Class I genes are HLA-A, -B and -C, and the class II locus is composed of several sub-regions that include the HLA-D antigens. These molecules are mainly expressed on B cells, macrophages and activated T-lymphocytes, but aberrant HLA expression may occur in certain autoimmune diseases. Class I antigens consist of two polypeptide sub-units, a heavy chain which is encoded within the major histocompatibility complex and microglobulin, which is a non-polymorphic polypeptide. The latter is encoded by a gene which maps to chromosome 15. The class II molecules are heterodimers, composed of two sub-units, both of which are encoded within the major histocompatibility complex.

The HLA-A alleles on a given chromosome are very closely linked, and are transmitted together as a haplotype. These alleles are co-dominant. Each parent has two haplotypes, both of which are expressed, and is able to transmit one or the other to each child. Parent and child will therefore share only one haplotype. HLA haplotypes show marked linkage disequilibrium.

The best described associations with class I genes are ankylosing spondylitis with HLA-B27, and 21-hydroxylase deficiency causing congenital adrenal hyperplasia with DW47. There are also associations between HLA-A3 and haemochromatosis, and psoriasis and the class I antigen CW6.

Narcolepsy and multiple sclerosis are associated with HLA-DR2, and many autoimmune diseases are DR3 associated, including SLE, in which the DR3 antigen commonly occurs in extended haplotype with the class I genes and A1 and B8, and the complement C4A null gene. Rheumatoid arthritis is most commonly associated with HLA-DR4, and not DR3.

126. (a) F.
    (b) F.
    (c) T.
    (d) T.
    (e) T.

Nimodipine is a calcium slow channel antagonist of the dihydropyridine class. A major site of action is at the sarcolemma, where it stabilises calcium channels in the inactive mode, producing a blockage of calcium entry. Nimodipine is most effective on arterioles with a diameter of < 100 μm, and is relatively selective for cerebral vessels. It may have a role in the prevention of delayed ischaemic neurological deficits from cerebral arterial spasm following sub-arachnoid haemorrhage.

Nizatidine is one of the many new H_2-receptor antagonists, used in the treatment of peptic ulcer disease. On a weight for weight basis it is around ten times more potent than cimetidine, but the drug has no H_1 antagonist activity.

The precise mode of action of omeprazole is still unclear, but its effects are largely thought to be mediated by specific binding to the parietal cell proton pump H^+- and K^+-ATPase located in the gastric mucosa. This enzyme is found on the apical membrane and in the tubular vesicles which lie in the secretory canniculi of the parietal cells. Omeprazole can decrease basal and stimulated gastric acid secretion independent of the stimulus.

Pamidronate is an amino-substituted geminal bisphosphonate, with very potent inhibitory effects on bone resorption mediated by osteoclasts. Its effect is demonstrable both *in vivo* and *in vitro*. The drug acts directly on the absorbing osteoclasts, and also inhibits the differentiation of precursor cells into mature osteoclasts. The drug is primarily indicated for the treatment of tumour-induced hypercalcaemia.

Acyclovir is an anti-viral agent which is two to three log orders more active against viral enzymes compared with their mammalian counterparts. The drug is phosphorylated by viral thymidine kinase to acyclovir monophosphate, and other enzymes convert this to the tri-phosphate metabolite of the drug. This is a potent inhibitor of DNA polymerase and prevents formation of viral DNA. GTP is incorporated into viral DNA, causing termination of biosynthesis. It is primarily used in the treatment of HSV and varicella zoster infection.

127. (a) T.
      (b) F.
      (c) F.
      (d) F.
      (e) T.

Nitric oxide is synthesised from L-arginine by nitric oxide synthases and three isoforms of nitric oxide synthase have been identified, an endothelial type, a neuronal type and a macrophage or inducible type. The cardiovascular system is actively dilated by nitric oxide, which inhibits adhesion and aggregation of platelets and white cells. It has been shown to be the active moiety of glyceryl trinitrate and has been shown to be deficient in some cases of essential hypertension.

128. (a) F.
    (b) F.
    (c) T.
    (d) F.
    (e) T.
Cefotaxime (and ceftriaxone) have little anti-pseudomonal activity, agents effective against pseudomonas include ceftazidime, piperacillin, imipenem, aminoglycosides and quinolones. Teicoplanin (and vancomycin) are only active against Gram-positive bacteria. Enterococci are resistant to all available cephalosporins. Clarithromycin is one of the more effective agents as part of combination therapy for atypical mycobacterial infections. Clindamycin has excellent activity against streptococci, staphylococci and anaerobes.

129. (a) T. The disease has complete penetrance but highly variable expressivity, even within a kindred.
    (b) T. The gene was cloned in 1990 by positional cloning methods (see above). It is very large, and includes several other genes within it, on the opposite strand.
    (c) T. Typical features are Café–au-lait spots, fibromatous skin tumours, Lisch nodules in the iris and there is is an increased risk of malignant tumours. Note that neurofibromatosis occurs in 5% of patients with phaeochromocytoma.
    (d) F. This condition displays one of the highest rates of new mutations of any disorder (about 50% patients are new mutants). This may be related to the size of the gene.
    (e) T. The reason for this observation is not known.

130. (a) F.
    (b) T.
    (c) F.
    (d) T.
    (e) T.
Deficiency of both serum and secretory IgA is the most common immunodeficiency. It occurs with a frequency of between 1:400 and 1:900 in various normal healthy populations. IgA deficiency is more prevalent among patients with

frequent infections, allergy and a range of autoimmune diseases including RA, SLE, Sjogren's, haemolytic anaemia, ITP and Addison's disease. There is also said to be an association with malignancies of the gastrointestinal tract, lymphomas, and malabsorption. Transient IgA deficiency is sometimes found in young children. This is generally less severe than the 'permanent' adult condition in which levels in serum are $< 0.05 \text{ g l}^{-1}$, and secretory IgA is undetectable. IgA deficiency can occur secondary to exposure to drugs such as penicillamine, phenytoin, and gold.

IgG sub-class deficiency occurs three times more frequently in boys than girls, but in adults there is a switch in the sex ratio. IgG sub-class deficiency is three times more common in women as in men. IgG2 deficiency is more common in children, and IgG3 deficiency in adults. IgG2 and IgG4 production is somewhat delayed during the normal development of the immune response in young children. In infancy there is often a poor response to polysaccharide antigens which mainly induce IgG2 antibodies, and in some children IgG1 antibodies are produced instead.

131. (a) T.
     (b) T.
     (c) F.
     (d) T.
     (e) T.

There are a number of cases of patients successfully treated by allogeneic bone marrow transplantation in the literature. In 1982 a young black American girl with acute myeloid leukaemia was treated in this manner, with cure of both her homozygous sickle cell disease and her leukaemia. At present, it is difficult to predict which patients are likely to experience a severe clinical course, and this combined with donor availability and cost mean that the procedure is unlikely to be used routinely in the immediate future. The genetic basis of the condition is well-characterised, and antenatal diagnosis can be performed on samples obtained at aminocentesis or chorionic villus sampling.

Proliferative sickle retinopathy is amenable to photocoagulation therapy. This complication is relatively common. In sickle cell haemoglobin C (SC disease) three-quarters of adults are affected by proliferative sickle retinopathy at some stage, but permanent visual loss occurs in 1:100 affected eyes.

The chronic compensated haemolytic anaemia of sickle disease increases the need for adequate dietary folate, and in certain populations, particularly in Africa, this may be lacking in the diet. Megaloblastic erythropoiesis may develop as a complication of folate shortage.

Hyposplenism is an important feature of sickle cell disease, and pneumococcal septicaemia may occur as a result. Penicillin prophylaxis is widely used in young children, who may respond poorly to pneumoccal vaccination before the age of 4 or 5 years.

132. (a) T.
  (b) T.
  (c) F.
  (d) F.
  (e) T.

Paget's disease affects up to 10% of patients over 70 years whilst only 5% are symptomatic. The disease is more common in males with a M:F ratio of 3:1. The most common presenting symptom is pain which may arise from a variety of sources including increased vascularity, periosteal distortion or from a site of mechanical stress. The disease is also associated with bony deformity and an increased incidence of secondary osteo-arthritis. In addition to clinical presentation a variety of investigations provide useful pointers to the diagnosis. These include scintigraphy which is a sensitive but non-specific way of assessing disease activity and distribution. Paget's disease is characterised by a combination of increased osteoclastic activity with osteoblastic remodelling. Typically the serum calcium, phosphate, parathyroid hormone, and vitamin D metabolites are all normal. However, the alkaline phosphatase and particularly bony alkaline phosphatase are typically raised and can be used to monitor disease activity whilst osteocalcin has proved disappointing in this regard. The development of potent antiresorptive drugs including the bisphosphonates etidronate, pamidronate and alendronate has produced a marked improvement in the treatment of this disease. High doses (> 10 mg kg^{-1} body weight) may result in defective bone mineralisation and, on occasions, fractures.

133. (a) F.
    (b) T.
    (c) F.
    (d) T.
    (e) T.

The granulocyte and granulocyte–macrophage colony stimulating factors (CSF) available for clinical use are products of recombinant DNA technology. The CSF are peptide hormones which are active in very small quantities and bind to specific receptors present on the surface of myeloid cells. The CSF have a short duration and are typically administered as a single daily subcutaneous injection which lasts for a few hours. They act to increase the number of stem cells in the circulation and shorten the time needed for their maturation into functionally competent cells. It is recommended that the CSF are not administered until 24 hours after the cessation of chemotherapy to avoid exposing precursor cells to damage from cytotoxic drugs. A number of indications for the use of these drugs exist including the treatment of neutropaenia after chemotherapy or ganciclovir treatment and the acceleration of myeloid recovery after bone-marrow transplantation. Reported serious side-effects are rare and may include fever, injection site reactions, myalgia and a capillary leak syndrome resulting in pulmonary oedema. These drugs are extremely powerful tools in the manipulation of haemopoesis and it is likely that further growth factors will be soon available. However, it should be borne in mind that the possibility of these agents themselves inducing haematological malignancies is not yet fully resolved and they should be used with caution under expert guidance.

134. (a) F.
    (b) F.
    (c) F.
    (d) T.
    (e) F.

The outer polysaccharide capsule is the major virulence factor of *S. pneumoniae* and immunity depends upon strain-specific anti-capsular antibodies. Therefore, the vaccine has to contain capsular antigen for each individual strain to confer immunity. There are over 80 capsular types of pneumococcus and currently the vaccine contains capsular antigen of the 23 most prominent pneumococcal serotypes. Patients with HIV have an increase in pneumococcal pneumonia and bacteraemia related to impaired specific antibody production. All HIV infected individuals should receive pneumococcal vaccination as early as possible as the antibody response to vaccines diminishes as HIV infection progresses. Penicillin resistance is an increasing problem, in the UK 1–2% of isolates are resistant but in parts of southern Europe the figure is 20–50%. Leukopenia is a grave prognostic sign in pneumococcal infections.

135. (a) T. Mutations in the *RET* gene have been described recently.
(b) T. Both MEN type 1 and type 2 are autosomal dominant disorders.
(c) T. Measurement of calcitonin, with or without a provocation test is useful for the detection of medullary thyroid cancer, in the detection of metastases, and the monitoring of therapy. Elevated plasma catecholamines may suggest the co-existence of a phaeochromocytoma.
(d) F. This is the frequency of pancreatic islet adenomas in MEN type I.
(e) F. Genetic screening by DNA analysis gives unambiguous results and often avoids the need for repetitive biochemical screening. It is particularly useful for analysis of 'at risk' family members in an affected kindred, who may comply poorly with regular biochemical screening.

136. (a) T.
(b) T.
(c) T.
(d) F.
(e) T.
Syndrome X is a term used by cardiologists as a diagnostic label in patients with angina who have a positive exercise test but normal coronary angiography. There is good evidence that coronary endothelial dysfunction is implicated in many patients, and the condition is associated with impaired EDRF activity.

Glucose tolerance tests in Syndrome X patients have been shown to be abnormal, and induce a hyperinsulinaemic response. Levels of pro-insulin and split products are elevated, as well as those of C-peptide, which is an indicator of insulin release from the pancreatic β-cells. It has been suggested that insulin resistance may be a consequence of impaired perfusion of the tissues, due to a loss of EDRF activity. The precise mechanistic links between insulin resistance, endothelial dysfunction, and so called microvascular angina remain to be fully elucidated. Pro-insulin and insulin are able to induce plasminogen activator inhibitor type 1 (PAI1), which reduces activation of TGF, a major regulator of extra-cellular matrix production and cellular growth.

137. (a) T.
  (b) F.
  (c) F.
  (d) T.
  (e) F.

Interferon-α is available in two main forms, a recombinant preparation, and as lymphoblastoid interferon which is a highly purified blend of natural human interferons, obtained from human lymphoblastoid cells following induction with Sendai virus. Interferon-α has been used in the therapy of hepatitis B and C in the chronic phase of the disease, hairy cell leukaemia, chronic myelogenous leukaemia, multiple myeloma, AIDS-related Kaposi's sarcoma, condylomata accuminata (by intra-lesional administration), and in the treatment of advanced non-Hodgkin's lymphoma in combination with an appropriate chemotherapeutic regimen.

The lymphoblastoid preparation is primarily indicated for the treatment of patients with hairy cell leukaemia. The drug is myelo-suppressive, and may affect leukocytes and platelets particularly, and is also associated with hypotension which may occur immediately after the administration of the drug, or one or two days later. Cardiac arrhythmias may result, and pulmonary infiltrates, pneumonia, or pneumonitis have been observed in interferon-treated patients. The drug may also affect the central nervous system, and cause depression and other psychiatric syndromes. Fever and flu-like symptoms are very common.

The mode of action of interferons is poorly understood. Their anti-viral effects are related partly to intra-cellular inhibition of nucleic acid synthesis and inhibition of protein synthesis and DNA replication in virus-infected cells. They increase MHC class I expression and antigen presentation and activate NK cells to kill virus-infected cells. IFN-γ is distinct and is produced by effector T cells mainly after induction of the adaptive immune response and have an immunostimulatory role in addition to inducing both MHC class I and class II expression. Interferon-α and -β have a common receptor, while interferon-γ interacts with a different receptor complex. There are several sub-classes of interferon-α, and viruses induce mainly interferon-α production by cells, whereas other mitogens such as phytohaemagglutinin and concanavalin-A stimulate interferon-γ production by T lymphocytes. Interferon-β is produced by fibroblasts in response to stimulation by viruses.

Recent trials have suggested that interferon-β-1b (a nonglycosylated interferon produced by recombinant methods) may have a role in the treatment of relapsing–remitting multiple sclerosis, and may reduce the frequency and degree of severity of clinical relapses in ambulatory patients with the disease. Use of this expensive drug is not widespread at present, and it remains to be established whether it represents a genuine breakthrough in the management of MS.

138. (a) T.
  (b) F.
  (c) T.
  (d) F.
  (e) T.

There have been numerous outbreaks of food poisoning due to consumption of raw milk cheese in Europe reported in recent times. *Listeria monocytogenes*, *Brucella melitensis*, various *Salmonella* species, notably *Salmonella paratyphi* and enterotoxigenic *E. coli* have all been implicated. The latter may cause haemolytic-uraemic syndrome. There is no obligation in the European Union for manufacturers to indicate that their products were made from unpasteurised cow's or goat's milk at present. Patients who are immunocompromised, on long-term corticosteroids, are debilitated, diabetic, or have cancer, are all more susceptible to enteric infections caused from eating cheese made from unpasteurised milk. However, in the absence of appropriate labelling, patients may not know which products to avoid.

Vomiting which develops within 1–8 hours of ingestion of a contaminated product is likely to be due to staphylococccal entertoxin, a protein with a molecular weight of 3.5×10^4, that is resistant to boiling for 30 minutes. The emetic affect of enterotoxin is the result of direct central nervous system stimulation. Diarrhoea may also develop, but there is generally rapid convalescence and no fever.

139. (a) T. Heterozygotes have elevated plasma LDL levels, and deposition of cholesterol in tendons, skin and arteries. Coronary artery disease develops in early middle age. Homozygotes are more severely affected and may develop severe coronary atheroma very young (<20 years; see (c) below).
(b) T. Plasma cholesterol levels in homozygotes may be greater than 15 mmol l^{-1}, and 8–13 mmol l^{-1} in heterozygotes. Triglycerides may be normal.
(c) T. There is a 50% risk of MI in heterozygous males by age 50 years.
(d) F. HMGCoA reductase inhibitors are the mainstay of treatment for this condition.
(e) T. Familial defective apo B may be clinically indistinguishable from familial hypercholesterolaemia. The overwhelming majority of mutations in familial defective Apo B are caused by a single base substitution in the codon for arginine 3500.

140. (a) F.
    (b) F.
    (c) F.
    (d) F.
    (e) T.
    gp120 on the outer membrane protein of HIV mediates binding to the CD4 molecule on the surface of T cells and gp41 mediates fusion with the cell membrane to allow virus entry. Infection of T cells may lead to fusion of cells to form syncytia but not granulomata and the typical histology is of a reactive lymph node. The long terminal repeat of HIV has NFkB binding sites and stimuli such as TNF-α that activate NFkB lead to increased viral replication. Following acute infection HIV viral load reduces but it does not enter a true latent period with continuing viral replication in lymphoid tissue. Activated T cells are much more easily infected *in vitro*.

141. (a) F. Introns, apart from their probable evolutionary functions, can contain enhancer elements and even hold genes.
    (b) T. The human genome comprises around 100 000 genes. Most DNA is single-copy (75%). Fifteen per cent of DNA is

repetitive and interspersed with genes and other single-copy DNA, while about 10% occurs in clusters of highly repetitive repeat sequences organised tandemly, called 'satellite DNAs'.
(c) T. The centiMorgan is the standard unit of genetic 'distance'.
(d) F. Pseudogenes are scattered widely throughout the genome and are frequently mutated copies of functional genes.
(e) T. These short tandem repeats are highly variable in the number of repeat units with which they are formed and they are therefore highly polymorphic. They are useful genetic markers.

142. (a) T.
    (b) T.
    (c) F.
    (d) F.
    (e) F.
Hyponatraemia in the acutely sick patient is frequently multifactorial. However, it may occur specifically in the contexts of over-hydration after surgery or the administration of chemotherapy, liver failure, renal failure, drug administration and cardiac failure. In a recent study examining 184 episodes of severe hyponatraemia in American and British hospital populations, three-quarters of patients had clouding of consciousness while severely hyponatraemic. Numerous other neurological complications were also reported, including transient hemiplegia, seizures, limb weakness, dysarthria, positive Babinsky signs, hallucinations and tremor. Psychosis was also reported, and 29% of the patients reported in this study died in hospital. It was thought that in only a minority of these was their death specifically attributable to the electrolyte disturbance. Correction of hyponatraemia has been associated with the development of central pontine myelinolysis. Cells in the brain initially respond to hyponatraemia by swelling, and this in itself may result in coma, herniation and death. As hyponatraemia develops, the brain responds by losing intracellular potassium, and later 'idiogenic osmoles' such as creatine and others are also lost to facilitate adaptation to the reduced tonicity of the extracellular environment. With rapid correction of hyponatraemia, intracellular potassium may be rapidly restored, but not so the other 'idiogenic osmoles'. A consequence of this may be that the extracellular compartment becomes hypertonic in relation to the intracellular department,

with resulting dehydration of the oligodendrocytes. Dehydration may then stimulate subsequent demyelination a few days later. There is increasing evidence that these complications are more common in patients in whom sodium is corrected too rapidly, and therapy should be directed specifically at correction of the underlying cause of the electrolyte disturbance, and it is now widely recommended that a rate of correction of less than 10 mmol l^{-1} per 24 hours be employed. It is rarely necessary to administer hypertonic saline, and conservative measures, such as fluid restriction, and the cessation of causative drugs, are often safer.

143. (a) T.
  (b) F.
  (c) T.
  (d) T.
  (e) T.

Hypocomplementaemic urticarial vasculitis is an auto-immune disorder resembling cutaneous LE. It is strongly associated with auto-antibodies to the collagenous part of the C1q molecule, and patients typically have a very low C4 and CH50. A positive ANA is found in only about 20% patients, however. Clinical features include a vasculitic rash which is typically urticarial in nature, angioedema, mononeuritides, and obstructive lung disease. The condition may respond to steroid therapy, and dapsone and anti-malarial drugs are also very useful. Anti-C1q antibodies are found in 20–30% of patients with SLE, and the main differential diagnoses in a patient with suspected HUVS and a low C4 level are lupus, C1 esterase inhibitor deficiency, and cryoglobulinaemia.

144. (a) T.
  (b) T.
  (c) T.
  (d) T.
  (e) F.

Oncogenes are those genes which are thought to be involved in the multi-step development of neoplasia. Some have been identified by characterisation of transforming sequences in oncogenic viruses ('v-onc'). Where homologous genes exist in vertebrate genomes, they are called cellular oncogenes ('c-onc'), or proto-oncogenes. They are normally small genes involved in the regulation of cellular processes and may encode growth factors, growth factor receptors, transcription factors and protein kinases. These genes are only oncogenic if they are activated in an aberrant way. No proto-oncogenes involved in the synthesis of complement proteins have been described.

145. (a) F.
    (b) T.
    (c) F.
    (d) T.
    (e) T.

Although cryoglobulinaemia may cause Raynaud's phenomenon, Raynaud's is very common in young women and is only rarely associated with the presence of a cryoglobulin. Cryoglobulinaemia may occur in SLE, rheumatoid arthritis, and Sjögren's syndrome, and is also associated with infections and lymphoproliferative disorders.

A very low C4 is typically detected but C3 levels are usually normal. Blood for cryoglobulin estimation should be taken into a plain tube and delivered to the laboratory at 37°C. Clotting is allowed to occur at this temperature, and after centrifugation and removal of the clot, the serum is left at 4°C for 3–5 days, and then inspected for the presence of a cryoprecipitate. A cryoglobulin may, however, precipitate at any temperature below body temperature, making cardiopulmonary bypass, and the cooling of a patient for cardiac surgery potentially hazardous.

There are three types of cryoglobulin:

Type 1 – monoclonal praproteins of IgG or IgM isotype. These typically occur in patients with myeloma, CLL, or Waldenström's.

Type 2 – these comprise a monoclonal rheumatoid factor, and are typically seen in mixed essential cryoglobulinaemia, but also in association with auto-immune or lymphoproliferative disorders.

Type 3 – 'mixed cryoglobulinaemia' comprising polyclonal IgG and/or IgM, and complement. This is also found in auto-immune disorders and in association with infections such as CMV, EBV, Kala-azar, infective endocarditis, and hepatitis B and C. Hepatitis-associated cryoglobulinaemia is particularly common in Southern Europe (especially in Italy and Greece).

146. (a) T.
     (b) F.
     (c) T.
     (d) T.
     (e) T.

Gastric acid is produced by parietal cells in the gastric mucosa. Acid secretion is generally lower in women than men, and varies considerably within the normal population. Numerous factors stimulate acid production including acetylcholine, histamine, circulating amino acids and a number of hormones, the most important of which is gastrin. This is produced by specialised cells, the G-cells which are scattered among the mucus cells of the pyloric glands. Gastrin occurs in numerous molecular sizes, and may be sulfated or non-sulfated. Pentagastrin, is a synthetic peptide that contains the terminal amino acids of the molecule. This was widely used as a stimulator for gastric acid secretion in diagnostic testing procedures. In the antral mucosa the main form of gastrin is the G17 variant, while in plasma the 34 amino acid molecule is found most commonly.

Secretion of acid by the parietal cells is under tight feedback hormonal control. Acid itself inhibits gastrin release, and when antral pH falls below 1.5 the release of this hormone is almost totally suppressed. Acid, fat, and high tonicity in the local environment in the intestinal lumen also inhibit gastric acid secretion. D-cells produce somatostatin which inhibits secretion of gastric by the G-cells.

There is evidence that acid secretion is increased in asymptomatic individuals who are *Helicobacter pylori*-positive, and the production of somatostatin, which inhibits acid production is also reduced in these patients, resulting in relative hypergastrinaemia, and enhanced acid production. Acid secretion can be stimulated by gastrin-releasing peptides, and there is evidence that the local level of mRNA for gastrin-releasing peptides is increased in *Helicobacter pylori*-positive subjects compared with normal controls.

Drugs such as omeprazole and lanzoprazole, which are protein pump inhibitors, are potent inhibitors of acid production, and are widely used in the treatment of oesophagitis and symptoms due to acid reflux. Increased gastric acid secretion is almost invariably found in patients with a history of duodenal ulceration, hence the adage 'no acid, no ulcer'.

147. (a) T.
     (b) T.
     (c) F.
     (d) T.
     (e) T.

Plasma aspartate transaminase, alanine transaminase and gamma glutamyl transferase are all markers of chronic alcohol abuse. Gamma GT (GGT) has a diagnostic sensitivity of 62% or hospitalised alcoholics, while ALT, AST, and MCV are all less sensitive. The specificity of gamma GT is around 80%. Plasma phosphate is not a marker in this condition.

There is a number of newer biochemical markers of alcohol abuse, including carbohydrate-deficient transferrin (CDT), mitochondrial AST (mAST) and alpha glutathione s-transferase. In a recent study AST, mAST and GGT were the best markers for distinguishing heavy alcohol usage from lower levels. The AST/ALT ratio may be useful in distinguishing alcohol abusers from patients with non-alcohol-related liver disease.

148. (a) T.
     (b) T.
     (c) F.
     (d) F.
     (e) T.

The oxidative modification of low density lipoproteins by free radicals is felt to be a major factor in the pathogenesis of atherosclerosis and it is also likely that oxidative damage to nucleic acids may have a key role in carcinogenesis. Natural enzymic anti-oxidants, the actions of which are complemented by various dietary anti-oxidant compounds control these processes. There is epidemiological evidence to link poor intake of dietary compounds of this type with increased risk of both cancer and ischaemic heart disease.

Anti-oxidants are mainly present in fruit and vegetables, and include α-tocopherol (vitamin E), β-carotene (a vitamin A precursor), and vitamin C (ascorbic acid). Flavonoids, e.g. quercetin, and myrecetin are natural polyphenolic compounds found particularly in apples, onions and red wine. They also have anti-oxidant properties and there is great contemporary interest in their role in the prevention of coronary heart disease, which at present remains unproven.

149. (a) F.
   (b) F.
   (c) F.
   (d) T.
   (e) F.
   Pork and human insulin preparations are similarly immuno-
   genic, while beef is more so. Human insulin may be prepared by
   enzymatic modification of pork insulin, in which case it is
   labelled 'emp', or using a biosynthetic technique, in bacteria or
   yeast. Preparations made in the former are marked 'prb', the
   latter 'pyr'. Insulins such as Human Insulatard, Humulin Zn or
   Humulin I have 'intermediate' pharmacodynamic profiles, with
   peak action at 2–6 hours and a potential to last for 24 hours.
   However, their onset of action may be rapid, comparable to that
   of short-acting 'soluble' type preparations, though may vary
   from 30 minutes to 3 hours. 'Mixtard' preparations are
   'biphasic' and may last up to 24 hours. They contain soluble
   insulin and have a rapid onset, and their subsequent
   pharmacodynamics depends on the proportion of soluble and
   isophane insulins in the preparation used.

   While multiple injection regimens are very popular, there is
   no firm evidence at present that they necessarily result in
   improved control, or fewer long-term complications than say,
   twice-daily regimens.

150. (a) F.
   (b) T.
   (c) F.
   (d) T.
   (e) F.
   Albumin, uric acid, urea and fasting blood glucose are generally
   lower in pregnancy than in non-pregnant control females, as of
   course, is the haemoglobin (especially in later pregnancy, due to
   the greatly expanded plasma volume). Plasma lipids, alkaline
   phosphatase, thyroxine binding globulin, and complement (C3
   and C4) levels all rise. Complement levels rise due to increased
   hepatic synthesis.

   Prednisolone at low dose, and at higher doses for short
   periods, is relatively safe in pregnancy. Placental 11β-dehy-
   drogenase metabolises both prednisolone and hydrocortisone to
   inactive keto forms, but not dexamethasone. Low-dose steroid

therapy is often preferable to NSAIDs in pregnancy in the management of inflammatory arthritis.

Antibodies to negatively-charged phospholipids, occurring in either primary antiphospholipid syndrome or SLE are associated with early abortion and also with late fetal damage due to placental insufficiency. However, in the absence of active renal disease, many patients with SLE sustain successful pregnancies, though monitoring in a specialist centre is needed. Post-delivery flares do occur, but can generally be controlled with appropriate modification in therapy (usually corticosteroids).

151. (a) F.
    (b) T.
    (c) F.
    (d) F.
    (e) F.

The nephrotic syndrome can be defined as the combination of proteinuria (>3.5 g 1.73 m^{-2} per day), hypoalbuminaemia (<30 g l^{-1}), and dependent oedema. Hypertension is a common associated finding in all patients except those with minimal change nephropathy (MCN). Hypercholesterolaemia is invariable and predisposes to accelerated atherosclerosis and may contribute to glomerular damage. Arterial and venous thromboses are common and effect in particular the deep veins of the leg and the renal veins. The patients also have an increased risk of infection which require early aggressive treatment. Attempts should be made to decrease the proteinuria and angiotensin converting-enzyme (ACE) inhibitors do this by reduction in the tone of the efferent arteriole which reduces pressure in the glomerular capillary. ACE inhibitors may reduce proteinuria by up to 50% if used in conjunction with salt restriction.

Minimal change nephropathy as a cause of nephrotic syndrome is particularly common in young children, whilst accounting for 20% of adult cases. Treatment with corticosteroids induces remission in 90% of cases within 3 weeks. Relapse is treated with further courses of treatment and if relapse is recurrent cyclophosphamide is indicated. Membranous nephropathy may be associated with hepatitis B, gold, penicilla-mine, malignancy and systemic lupus erythematosus. Approximately 40% of patients undergo spontaneous remission within 5 years.

152. (a) T.
     (b) T.
     (c) T.
     (d) T.
     (e) T.

Infectious mononucleosis complications include splenic rupture, myocarditis, pericarditis, polyneuritis, cranial nerve palsies, meningitis, encephalitis, transverse myelitis, interstitial nephritis, glomerulonephritis, pharyngeal oedema and respiratory obstruction, arthritis, haemolysis, agranulocytosis, agammaglobulinaemia and thrombocytopaenia.

NB. The Paul–Bunnell test for heterophile antibody against sheep red cells, unabsorbed serum and guinea-pig absorbed serum are positive while Ox absorbed serum is negative.

153. (a) T.
     (b) T.
     (c) F.
     (d) T.
     (e) T.

Hereditary non-polyposis colon cancer is the commonest form of inherted colonic cancer. The condition is defined by the occurrence of colon cancer in three family members (two of whom must be first degree relatives). Two generations must be affected, with one subject diagnosed with a colonic tumour under 50 years of age. A 'replication error' (RER) phenotype is seen in HNPCC individuals. Tumour DNA contains aberrant microsatellite alleles not seen in DNA from the patient's normal tissues. Five 'mis-match repair' (MMR) genes have now been found in man, and germline mutations in four of these have been described in HNPCC patients. Other MMR genes may yet be found. Extra-colonic tumours may also occur in HNPCC patients (e.g. stomach, uterine endometrium, and ovary).

Half the families with inherited breast carcinoma have mutations in the *BRCA1* gene. These patients may also have ovarian cancers. A second gene *BRCA2* has also been found recently which may be responsible for many of the remaining inherited breast cancers in women, and many inherited male breast cancers.

154. (a) T.
     (b) T.

(c) T.
(d) T.
(e) T.
Growth hormone (GH) has a key role in somatic development. It exerts its effects on tissues in a number of ways, one of which is *via* the induction of insulin-like growth factor 1 (IGF-1). This has marked trophic effect on muscle cells, and can induce transcription of a number of genes such as myosin light-chain-2, troponin I and skeletal muscle α-actin. In the heart, IGF-1 mRNA increases with pressure overload, and is markedly elevated in ventricular hypertrophy. Cardiac failure developing due to dilated cardiomyopathy in a number of patients with hypopituitarism has been successfully treated with GH, and this raises the possibility that GH may be useful generally in the treatment of heart failure due to dilated cardiomyopathy, in which there is ventricular dilation, in the absence of an adequate increase in wall thickness. Recombinant GH is the treatment of choice in deficient children, and has many attractions for athletes and body builders, in view of the difficulty of detecting its exogenous administration.

155. (a) F.
      (b) T.
      (c) T.
      (d) T.
      (e) T.
Lesch–Nyhan syndrome is indeed due to a defect in purine metabolism due to deficiency of hypoxanthine guanine phosphoribosyl transferase, but the disorder is X-linked, resulting in gout, spasticity, choreoathetosis, mental retardation and self-mutilation.

Tay–Sachs disease is a G_{M2} gangliosidosis due to a genetic defect in hexosaminidase A, an enzyme which is the product of a 3-gene system encoding an activator protein and α and β subunits of the enzyme. The disease affects the CNS and causes progressive neurological deterioration between the age of 3 months until death, 2–3 years later. About 1:30 Ashkenazi Jews carry the Tay–Sachs allele.

Hurler and Hunter syndromes are mucopolysaccharidoses, a group of disorders which are due to defects in enzymes responsible for the physiological degradation of glycosamino-glycans. Hurler syndrome is autosomal recessive, and results in corneal clouding, 'gargoyl' facies, skeletal abnormalities, hydrocephalus, hepatosplenomegaly, mental retardation and death before puberty. Hunter syndrome has a milder phenotype and is X-linked recessive. Most enzymopathies are recessive, as heterozygotes make around 50% normal product, which is usually enough, except in situations where the enzyme is a rate-limiting factor in a cascade (e.g. in the synthesis of porphyrins). α_1-Anti-trypsin deficiency represents an excellent example of the interaction of genes and environmental factors in pathogenesis. Patients with the common Z/Z genotype, who develop emphysema and cirrhosis, have a worse prognosis after the age of 60 if they smoke. This has been attributed to the fact that the active site of the enzyme, at methionine 358, is readily oxidised by compounds in cigarette smoke, with a 3 log resultant reduction in its affinity for elastase.